Overtime and Extended Work Shifts:
Recent Findings on Illnesses, Injuries, and Health Behaviors

Claire C. Caruso, Ph.D., R.N.
Edward M. Hitchcock, Ph.D.
Robert B. Dick, Ph.D.
John M. Russo, Ph.D.
Jennifer M. Schmit, M.A.

U. S. Department of Health and Human Services
Centers for Disease Control and Prevention
National Institute for Occupational Safety and Health

Ordering Information

To receive documents or other information about occupational safety and health topics, contact the National Institute for Occupational Safety and Health (NIOSH) at

NIOSH Publications Dissemination
4676 Columbia Parkway
Cincinnati, OH 45226-1998

Telephone: 1-800-35-NIOSH (1-800-356-4674)
Fax: 1-513-533-8573
E-mail: pubstaft@cdc.gov
or visit the NIOSH Web site at www.cdc.gov/niosh

DHHS (NIOSH) Publication No. 2004-143

Foreword

The average number of hours worked annually by workers in the United States has increased steadily over the past several decades and currently surpasses that of Japan and most of Western Europe. The influence of overtime and extended work shifts on worker health and safety, as well as on worker errors, is gaining increased attention from the scientific community, labor representatives, and industry. U.S. hours of service limits have been regulated for the transportation sector for many years. In recent years, a number of states have been considering legislation to limit mandatory overtime for health care workers. The volume of legislative activity seen nationwide indicates a heightened level of societal concern and the timeliness of the issue.

This document summarizes recent scientific findings concerning the relationship between overtime and extended work shifts on worker health and safety. The number of studies increased dramatically over the past few years, but important research questions remain. I am confident that this document will contribute to an informed discussion of these issues and provide a basis for further research and analysis.

John Howard, M.D.
Director,
National Institute for Occupational Safety and Health

Executive Summary

PURPOSE

This report provides an integrative review of 52 recently published research reports that examine the associations between long working hours and illnesses, injuries, health behaviors, and performance. The report is restricted to a description of the findings and methods and is not intended as an exhaustive discussion of all important issues related to long working hours. Findings and methods are summarized as reported by the original authors, and the study methods are not critically evaluated for quality.

SUMMARY

In 16 of 22 studies addressing general health effects, overtime was associated with poorer perceived general health, increased injury rates, more illnesses, or increased mortality. One meta-analysis of long work hours suggested a possible weak relationship with preterm birth. Overtime was associated with unhealthy weight gain in two studies, increased alcohol use in two of three studies, increased smoking in one of two studies, and poorer neuropsychological test performance in one study. Some reports did not support this trend, finding no relationship between long work hours and leisure-time physical activity (two of three studies) and no relationship with drug abuse (one study).

A pattern of deteriorating performance on psychophysiological tests as well as injuries while working long hours was observed across study findings, particularly with very long shifts and when 12-hour shifts combined with more than 40 hours of work a week. Four studies that focused on effects during extended shifts reported that the 9th to 12th hours of work were associated with feelings of decreased alertness and increased fatigue, lower cognitive function, declines in

vigilance on task measures, and increased injuries. Two studies examining physicians who worked very long shifts reported deterioration on various measures of cognitive performance.

When 12-hour shifts combined with other work-related demands, a pattern of more adverse findings was detected across studies. Six studies examining 12-hour shifts combined with more than 40 hours of work per week reported increases in health complaints, deterioration in performance, or slower pace of work. Two studies comparing 8- and 12-hour schedules during day and night shifts reported that 12-hour night shifts were associated with more physical fatigue, smoking, or alcohol use. Two studies examining start times for 12-hour shifts reported that decrements in alertness or more health complaints were associated with early 6:00 a.m. start times. One study examining 12-hour shifts in hot work environments reported a slower pace of work as compared with shorter shifts. Another study examining high workloads during 12-hour shifts showed increased discomfort and deterioration in performance as compared with shorter shifts.

More definitive statements about differences between 8-hour and 12-hour shifts are difficult because of the inconsistencies in the types of work schedules examined across studies. Work schedules differed by the time of day (i.e., day, evening, night), fixed versus rotating schedules, speed of rotation, direction of rotation, number of hours worked per week, number of consecutive days worked, number of rest days, and number of weekends off. All of these factors could have interacted with overtime and influenced study results. Also, some studies did not report how many hours participants worked per week or other details about the work shifts, which complicated the assessment of their results. The many differences in the 8- and 12-hour shift schedules studied may have accounted for their contradictory findings.

Few studies have examined related topics, such as the combined influence of shift work and overtime, or how worker control over their work time and mandatory overtime might influence their health.

Some studies examined functional abilities or injuries during the 1st to 12th hours of work, but little has been reported about effects after the 12th hour. Few studies have investigated the influence of long working hours on the health and safety of women or older workers. Few studies have explored how long working hours influence workers with pre-existing health problems, or how the hours relate to symptom management and the course of common chronic diseases. Little data are available regarding the influence of occupational exposures (i.e., chemical, heat, noise, lifting) in combination with long working hours on health and safety.

Although the number of published studies examining long working hours appears to be increasing, many research questions remain on how overtime and extended work shifts influence worker health and safety.

Table of Contents

Foreword. iii

Executive Summary iv

Tables viii

Abbreviations. ix

Acknowledgments. x

1. Introduction. 1

2. Description of the Work Schedules and the Samples. 3

3. Health and Safety Findings 5

    3.1 Findings Associated with Overtime. 5
        3.1a Overtime and Cardiovascular Findings. 5
        3.1b Overtime and Other Illnesses. 8
        3.1c Overtime and Injuries 12
        3.1d Overtime and Health Behaviors 12
        3.1e Overtime and Performance. 12

    3.2 Findings Associated with Extended Work Shifts 12
        3.2a Extended Work Shifts and Illnesses. 17
        3.2b Extended Work Shifts and Injuries. 17
        3.2c Extended Work Shifts and Health Behaviors. 17
        3.2d Extended Work Shifts and Performance 17

    3.3 Findings Associated with Extended Work Shifts Combined with More than 40-Hours
        Work per Week 21
        3.3a Extended Work Shifts Combined with More than 40-Hours Work per Week
            and Illnesses 21
        3.3b Extended Work Shifts Combined with More than 40-Hours Work per Week
            and Injuries 24
        3.3c Extended Work Shifts Combined with More than 40-Hours Work per Week
            and Health Behaviors 24
        3.3d Extended Work Shifts Combined with More than 40-Hours Work per Week
            and Performance 24

    3.4 Findings Associated with Very Long Shifts 24

      3.4a Very Long Shifts and Other Illnesses. 24
      3.4b Very Long Shifts and Performance 24

4. Summary 27
    4.1 Overtime 27
    4.2 Extended Work Shifts 27
    4.3 Other Work Schedule Characteristics. 28
    4.4 Compensation, Vacation Time, Commute Time 28
    4.5 Gender and Age 28
    4.6 Chronic Health Problems. 28
    4.7 Occupational Exposures. 29

5. Concluding Remarks 30

References 31

Tables

Table 1. Countries Where Studies Were Conducted 4

Table 2. Types of Work Investigated 4

Table 3. Studies Examining Overtime and Cardiovascular Outcomes: Methods and Findings 6

Table 4. Studies Examining Overtime and Other Illnesses: Methods and Findings 9

Table 5. Studies Examining Overtime and Injuries: Methods and Findings 13

Table 6. Studies Examining Overtime, Health Behaviors, and Performance Outcomes: Methods and
Findings 14

Table 7. Studies Examining Extended Work Shifts: Methods and Findings 18

Table 8. Studies Examining Extended Work Shifts Combined with More than 40 Hours per week:
Methods and Findings 22

Table 9. Studies Examining Very Long Work Shifts: Methods and Findings 25

Abbreviations

ANOVA	analysis of variance
ANOCOVA	analysis of covariance
BMI	body mass index
BP	blood pressure
CI	confidence interval
CIR	cumulative incidence ratio
D	day
DART	Division of Applied Research and Technology
E	evening
h	hour
M	mean
N	night
NIOSH	National Institute for Occupational Safety and Health
NS	not significant
OR	odds ratio
OSHA	Occupational Safety and Health Administration
PR	prevalence risk ratio
R	range
RR	relative risk ratio
wk	week
y	years

Acknowledgments

The following contributors are gratefully acknowledged for their efforts on this document: Roger R. Rosa, Ph.D. (NIOSH, Office of the Director, Senior Scientist), Steven L. Sauter, Ph.D. (NIOSH, Division of Applied Research and Technology (DART), Chief, Organizational Sciences and Human Factors Branch), Thomas R. Waters, Ph.D., C.P.E. (NIOSH, DART, Supervisory Industrial Engineer), and B.K. Nelson, Ph.D. (NIOSH, DART, Research Toxicologist).

Editorial review by Anne L. Votaw, Writer/Editor, NIOSH, DART.
Document layout by Brenda J. Jones, Visual Information Specialist, NIOSH, DART.

Credits for cover photos:

>   *Nighttime Lights of the USA*. Satellite imagery: U.S. Air Force and the National Oceanic and Atmospheric Administration.
>
>   Foundry worker and assembly worker: Parker D.L. [2002]. *By These Hands*. St. Paul, MN: Minnesota Historical Society Press.
>
>   Medical worker: http://www.corbis.com.
>
>   Worker at a computer: Brenda Jones, Visual Information Specialist, NIOSH, DART.

We thank the following external reviewers of this document.

Alison Trinkoff, Sc.D., R.N., F.A.A.N.
Professor
School of Nursing
University of Maryland
655 West Lombard
Baltimore, MD 21201

Timothy Monk, Ph.D.
Clinical Neuroscience Research Center
Western Psychiatric Institute and Clinic
University of Pittsburgh Medical Center
TDH E1123 Pittsburgh
Pittsburgh, PA 15213

Bill Kojola
Department of Occupational Safety and Health
AFL-CIO (American Federation of Labor - Congress of Industrial Organizations)
815 16th St. NW
Washington, DC 20006

Gordon Smith, M.D., M.P.H.
Yueng-Hsiang (Emily) Huang, Ph.D.
Center for Safety Research
Liberty Mutual Research Center for Safety & Health
71 Frankland Road
Hopkinton, MA 01748

> The annual number of hours worked per person in the United States surpasses Japan and most of Western Europe.
>
> *[International Labour Office 2002]*

1. Introduction

Overtime is common in the United States and has increased steadily from 1970 through the 1990s [Hetrick 2000; Rones et al. 1997]. According to the International Labour Office [2002], the annual number of hours worked per person in the United States surpasses Japan and most of Western Europe. Figure 1 displays the average annual work hours for the locations of studies discussed in this document [International Labour Office 2003]. As illustrated, work hours in the United States are only surpassed by Thailand, Hong Kong, and South Korea.

This document provides an integrative review of selected health and safety issues associated with overtime and extended work shifts. Findings are summarized as reported by the original authors, and the study methods are described, but not crit-

ically evaluated. For this document, *overtime* is defined as more than 40 hours per week and *extended work shifts* are defined as shifts longer than 8 hours.

Seventy-five research reports, including one meta-analysis, were identified according to the following criteria:

1. Focused on overtime or extended work shifts
2. Published from 1995 through 2002
3. Peer-reviewed publication
4. Published in the English language

The information retrieval databases used to identify reports include *Medline*, *Current Contents*, *PsycINFO*, and *ScienceDirect*. Keywords used in the search were *overtime, extended work shifts,*

Figure 1. Average Annual Work Hours by Country *[International Labour Office 2003]*

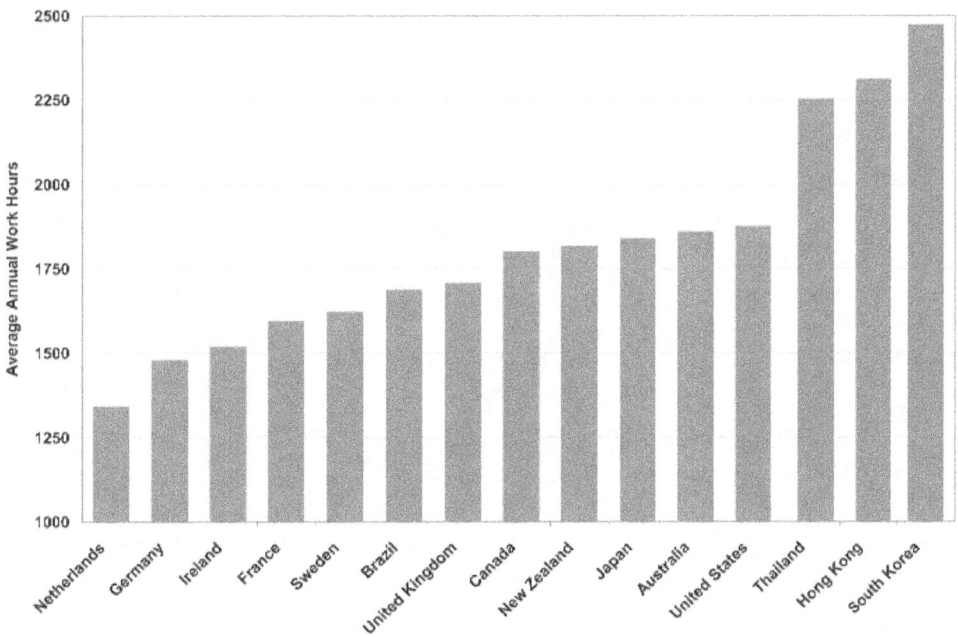

work hours, work schedule tolerance, 12-hour shifts, 10-hour shifts. Additionally, the references cited in the retrieved reports were examined for any relevant research reports. The studies examined a variety of health and safety issues, ranging from illnesses and injuries to social life and job satisfaction. The present report is limited to a summary of those studies that addressed associations between long working hours and illnesses, injuries, health behaviors, and performance. The health behaviors include physical activity, smoking, alcohol use, and body weight. Performance measures include automobile crashes, tests of cognitive functioning, executive functioning, subjective alertness, cardiovascular fatigue, and muscle fatigue. Of the 75* reports examined, 51 studies and one meta-analysis addressed these outcomes and are summarized below. The summary of findings does not include the remaining 23 reports that did not examine illnesses, injuries, health behaviors, or performance.

*Note: The papers not discussed in this document are indicated in the Reference section by ‡.

2. Description of the Work Schedules and the Samples

To examine the relationship of overtime and extended work shifts on health and safety, 52 research studies were classified under four categories, based on the information contained in the reports:

1. *Overtime*: most studies compared the number of hours worked by full-time participants and reported no other work schedule details.

2. *Extended work shifts:* 10- or 12-hour shifts were compared with 8-hour shifts in most studies and used a standard 40-hour work week. Some studies, however, did not clearly report the number of hours worked per week. Some studies, however, did not clearly report the number of hours worked per week.

3. *Extended work shifts combined with more than 40 hours per week*: 12-hour shifts compared with 8-hour shifts in most studies.

4. *Very long shifts* (e.g., resident physician on 32-hour call schedule and 48-hour taxi driver schedule).

The process of classifying the studies into these categories often was hampered by lack of a complete and clear description of the work schedules. For example, the studies examining 12-hour work shifts did not always clearly report the number of hours worked per week. Thus, some misclassification of studies is possible in this summary document. In addition, the complexity and wide variety of work schedules studied made it difficult to compare and synthesize findings across the 52 reports.

Work schedules differ in many ways, and more than 10,000 schedules are in use worldwide [Knauth 1998]. Time of work (day, evening, night), fixed or rotating shift, the degree of worker control over work times, number of hours worked per day, number of consecutive workdays before rest days, number of hours worked per week, number of rest days, and number of weekends off were all factors that combined in a variety of ways across these field studies. An individual study's finding for shift length or number of hours worked per week may have been influenced by time of work or other characteristics of the work schedule. Thus, some caution should be exercised in characterizing some of these studies or interpreting their findings solely in terms of long hours of work or extended shifts.

Tables 1 and 2 list the country where the studies were conducted and the type of work. Approximately 20% of the studies were conducted in the United States, 28% in Asia, and 35% in Europe. The studies were conducted in field settings, except for three laboratory investigations. The most frequent types of work studied were health care, *white collar*, and manufacturing. The age groups studied ranged from young adults to older workers in their 60s, but only two studies specifically addressed the relationship of age to health effects. Men were examined exclusively in 40% of the studies, as compared with 10% of studies that examined only women.

> Work schedules differ in many ways, and more than 10,000 schedules are in use worldwide.
>
> *[Knauth 1998]*

Table 1.
Countries Where Studies Were Conducted

Location	N
Asia	21
Australia	7
Canada	3
Europe	26
South America	1
United States	14
United States and Canada	1
United States and Europe	1
More than Two Locations	1

Note. Table covers all 75 publications examined.

Table 2.
Types of Work Investigated

Type of Work	N
Construction	2
Health Care	19
Manufacturing	21
Mining	2
Public Administration and Services	11
Transportation	3
Utilities	5
White Collar Work	24
Not Specified	12

Note. Table covers all 75 publications examined. Frequency counts will not sum to total number of publications, as some publications used multiple work types.

3. Health and Safety Findings

A summary of the findings for cardiovascular diseases and other illnesses, injuries, health behaviors, and performance effects are listed below. Findings are discussed for each of the four work schedule categories listed earlier.

3.1 FINDINGS ASSOCIATED WITH OVERTIME

Twenty-nine studies and one meta-analysis examined associations between overtime and the outcomes targeted for this report. The studies were conducted in Japan (10), United States (5), Sweden (5), Germany (2), South Korea (2), Canada (1), Hong Kong (1), Netherlands (1), Thailand (1), and United Kingdom (1). The studies used a variety of criteria to group participants based on the number of hours worked. For example, the criterion used to define the group with the lowest number of hours worked ranged widely from 35 to 60 hours per week across studies.

3.1a Overtime and Cardiovascular Findings

Table 3 displays the methods and results for the studies examining overtime and cardiovascular findings. Two case-control studies of Japanese workers reported that overtime during the previous month was associated with an increased risk for acute myocardial infarction. Liu et al. [2002] reported that 61 or more hours of work per week and less than 2 days off a month increased the

odds by two-fold or more. Sokejima and Kagamimori [1998] observed a U-shaped relationship: as compared with 7 to 9 hours of work per day, higher risk was associated with both shorter hours (less than 7 hours a day) and longer hours (more than 11 hours a day).

Findings for hypertension were inconsistent across four studies. Iwasaki et al. [1998] reported significantly *elevated* systolic blood pressure in older salesmen (ages 50 – 60) whose combined commute and work hours exceeded 61 hours per week as compared with older salesmen working 57 hours or less. No differences were reported in younger workers (ages 20 – 49 years). Hayashi et al. [1996] observed *increased* blood pressure in groups of *white collar* employees working 84 to 96 mean hours of overtime per month as compared with those working 25 to 43 mean hours of overtime. Nakanishi et al. [2001b], however, published the opposite results: *white collar* workers reporting 10 or more hours of work per day had a *lower* risk for developing hypertension when compared with workers reporting less than 8 hours of work per day. Lastly, Park et al. [2001a] reported no correlation between blood pressure and work hours in Korean engineers whose work hours during the previous month ranged from an average of 52 hours to 89 hours per week. No participants in this study worked less than 52 hours on average per week.

Table 3. Studies Examining Overtime and Cardiovascular Outcomes: Methods and Findings

Author, Date	Sample	Measure of Overtime	Cardiovascular Measure	Statistical Methods Controls	Results Reported By Authors
Hayashi et al.1996	Compared three groups of male *white collar* workers at one electronics plant: • Group sizes: 10 – 19 • Group M ages 36 – 47 • Japan	One month daily diary of work hours (overtime hours/month by group): • Comparison 1 with normal BP: ○ High overtime: 88 +/- 42 ○ Low overtime: 25 +/- 7 • Comparison 2 with elevated BP: ○ High overtime: 84 +/- 42 ○ Low overtime: 26 +/- 7 • Comparison 3 with workers examined twice during busy and slow season: ○ High overtime: 96 +/- 28 ○ Low overtime: 43 +/- 18	24-h blood pressure and heart rate measured every hour with portable monitor: • Normal BP: systolic < 140; diastolic < 85 • Elevated BP: systolic >140 to <160; diastolic > 90 to < 105	• t-test for independent samples tested the repeated measures of BP and pulse readings • Paired t-test tested seasonal group	• In Comparison 1 with normal BP, high overtime showed: ○ Higher average systolic and diastolic BP ○ Heart rate NS • In Comparison 2 with elevated BP, high overtime showed: ○ Higher average diastolic BP and heart rate ○ Systolic BP NS • In Comparison 3, workers during busy season showed: ○ Higher average systolic and diastolic BP ○ Higher heart rates
Iwasaki et al.1998	71 salesmen: • Age R 22 – 60 • Japan	One-time survey*: • Short work hours—57 h/wk • Long work hours—61 to 68 h/wk *Work hours defined as hours in office plus commute time during last month.	During one evening measured mean of two blood pressure readings.	t-test	Mean systolic blood pressure elevated for long-hour group as compared with short-hour group for ages 50 – 60, and no difference noted for ages 20 – 49.
Liu et al.2001	• 260 men with acute myocardial infarction (AMI) • 445 male controls • Age R 40 – 79 • *White collar and blue collar* workers • Japan	One-time interview: • Work h/wk: ≤ 40; 41 – 60; ≥ 61 • Days off/month: < 2; 2 – 7; ≥ 8 • Rotating shifts yes/no • Interactions: work hours and sleep length; work hours and days off/month	• Hospital records identified cases with AMI who survived to receive rehabilitation from 1996 to 1998. • Controls free of AMI: resident registers used to match for age, sex, residence. • Other measures: ○ Workday sleep hours: ≤ 5; 6 – 8; ≥ 9 ○ Days off sleep hours: ≤ 5; 6 – 8; ≥ 9 h ○ Days/wk with < 5h sleep	• ANOVA • ANACOVA • Logistic regression analysis: interaction of sleep with working hours assessed with likelihood ratio test. • Covariates: hypertension, diabetes, hyperlipidaemia, overweight, cigarette smoking, parental coronary heart disease, *blue collar/white collar job*, sedentary job	• Working > 61 h/wk increased risk by two fold for AMI compared with ≤40 h (CI 1.1 – 3.5). • < 2 days off in previous month increased risk (OR 2.9; CI 1.3 – 6.5). • Categories of longer work and less days off or short sleep time showed trend for increase in the OR, but none of interactions were significant.
Nakanishi et al. 2001b	941 male *white collar* workers from one building contractor: • No history of hypertension (HTN) • Age R 35 – 54 • Japan	Interview in 1994: work h/day < 8.0; 8.0 – 8.9; 9 – 9.9; 10.0 – 10.9; ≥ 11.0 h/wk	• BP measurements during annual health exam from 1994 to 1999 • World Health Organization criteria for HTN: ○ Systolic blood pressure ≥ 160 mm Hg ○ Diastolic blood pressure ≥ 95 mm Hg ○ Taking BP medication	• ANOVA • Cox proportional hazard method: covariates (measured 1994): age, occupation, position, BMI, alcohol intake, commute time, vegetable and salt intake, eating breakfast, smoking, exercise, sleep length.	• 336 men developed borderline HTN or definite HTN. • 88 men developed definite HTN. • Relative risk for borderline HTN or definite HTN (reference category < 8 h/day): ○ 10 – 10.9 h/day .63 (CI 1.43 – .91) ○ >11.0 h/day .48 (CI .31 – .74) • Relative Risk for definite HTN: >11h/day .33 (CI .11 – .95)
Park et al. 2001a	238 male engineers from 3 electronics manufacturing plants: • Age M 32, R 22 – 46 • South Korea	One-time questionnaire: M h/wk during previous month (R 52 – 89 h/wk)	Blood pressure on afternoon of the survey day	• Correlation coefficients • Multiple linear regression • Covariates: age and hours of sleep	Weekly working hours showed no significant correlation with blood pressure.

Table 3. Studies Examining Overtime and Cardiovascular Outcomes: Methods and Findings (Continued)

Author, Date	Sample	Measure of Overtime	Cardiovascular Measure	Statistical Methods Controls	Results Reported By Authors
Sokejima and Kagamimori 1998	195 men (age M 55) with first acute myocardial infarction (AMI) and 331 controls (age M 54): • 51% managers • 49% other occupations • Japan	Self-administered survey: • M work h/day for each of 2 months before AMI from cases or before enrollment into study from controls • M work h/day for the months with the shortest and longest mean work hours during previous year	• AMI cases established from hospital records • Control cases with no coronary artery disease from workplace medical exam • Matched for age and occupation	• Logistic regression • Covariates: age, occupation category, hypertension, hypercholesterolaemia, diabetes, body mass index, smoking habits, proportion of sedentary work, and burnout index	Hours worked during previous month showed U-shaped relationship. Higher risk for AMI associated with shorter hours ($\leq$ 7h/day; OR 2.8, CI 1.5 – 5.3) and longer hours (>11h/day; OR 2.9, CI 1.4 – 6.3) as compared with the reference category of (>7 – 9 h/day).

Note. Abbreviations used: BMI = body mass index; BP = blood pressure; CI = 95% confidence interval; CIR = cumulative incidence ratio; D = day; E = evening; h = hours; M = mean; N = night; NS = not significant; OR = odds ratio; PR = prevalence risk ratio; R = range; RR = relative risk ratio; wk = week; y = years.

3.1b Overtime and Other Illnesses

Table 4 displays the methods and results for the studies examining overtime and other illnesses. Overtime was associated with poorer perceived general health in three of four studies [Ettner and Grzywacz 2001; Kirkcaldy et al. 2000; Siu and Donald 1995; Worrall and Cooper 1999], increased neck or musculoskeletal discomfort in two studies [Bergqvist et al. 1995; Fredriksson et al. 1999], increased mortality in one study [Nylén et al. 2001], and subfecundity in one study [Tuntiseranee et al. 1998].

Mozurkewich et al. [2000] conducted a meta-analysis of 10 studies published between 1987 and 1997 and reported no association between long work hours and preterm birth. Further analysis of the six higher quality studies suggested a weak relationship between long working hours and preterm birth (Odd Ratio = 1.24 with a 95% Confidence Interval of 1.04 to 1.48). In contrast, Voss et al. [2001] reported that more than 50 hours of overtime during the previous year was associated with *less* sick time in a Swedish study.

Associations with diabetes mellitus in two Japanese prospective health studies were contradictory. Kawakami et al. [1999] reported that 50 or more hours of overtime per month *increased* the risk for development of diabetes mellitus as compared with 25 hours or less. In contrast, Nakanishi et al. [2001a] reported that 11 hours or more a day was associated with a *reduced* risk as compared with less than 8 hours. Both studies collected work hour data at the initial contact and did not examine the influence of working long hours over the course of several years.

In summary, overtime was associated with increased morbidity and mortality in 8 of 12 studies, and one meta-analysis suggested a possible weak relationship between overtime and preterm birth.

Combined relationship of pressure to work overtime and rewards in Dutch postal workers was examined by van der Hulst et al. [2001]. Rewards included salary, job security, and career opportunities. They reported that high pressure to work overtime in combination with low rewards was associated with a 3-fold increase in the odds for somatic complaints as compared with a reference category of low overtime pressure in combination with high rewards. In contrast, high pressure in combination with high rewards did not differ from the reference category. Ninety-five percent of the sample worked less than 50 hours per week.

Siu and Donald [1995] also reported a relationship with overtime pay. Men from Hong Kong who received no payment for overtime reported more health complaints when compared with men who received payment.

Mizoue et al. [2001] examined the relationship of overtime and sick building syndrome among Japanese municipal employees working in an environment with few workplace smoking restrictions. Thirty hours of overtime or more during the previous month was associated with a 2.6-fold increased risk for symptoms of general malaise and irritation of the mucous membranes and skin.

Fredriksson et al. [1999] examined the combined influence of domestic workload and overtime in workers from a broad range of occupations in Sweden. Additional domestic workload increased the cumulative incidence or prevalence risk for disorders of the neck in men and women who were working overtime.

Table 4. Studies Examining Overtime and Other Illnesses: Methods and Findings

Author, Date	Sample	Measure of Overtime	Other Illness Measure	Statistical Methods Controls	Results Reported By Authors
Bergquist et al. 1995	260 visual display terminal workers: • Women 76% • Sweden	One-time questionnaire: frequent overtime yes/no	One-time *Nordic Survey of Musculoskeletal Symptoms* and physiotherapeutic examination identified discomfort of arm/hand, neck/shoulder, back	• Multivariate logistic regression • Covariates: age, activities, attitudes, eye conditions, organization type, time planning, work load, ergonomic factors	Arm/hand discomforts associated with extensive overtime (OR 2.2, CI 1.2 – 4.4)
Ettner and Grzywacz 2001	Data from the 1995 mid-life study of 2,048 residents: • Age R 25 – 74, M 42 • Women 51% • United States	One-time questionnaire: average h/wk working at all jobs < 35, 35 – 45, >45	Combined responses from two questions asking effect of job on physical or emotional/mental health: 1 = negative; 2 = mixed; 3 = positive	• Ordinal logistic regression • Covariates: demographics, personality type, job characteristics	Working >45 h/wk increased by 25% likelihood of reporting negative effects of work on health
Fredriksson et al. 1999	484 *white collar* and *blue collar* workers from broad range of occupations without musculoskeletal diagnoses in 1969: • Age M 48, R 42 – 59 • Women 52% • Sweden	Interview in 1969: • Overtime yes/no (work hour criteria not specified) • Day versus night or shift work • Interactions: overtime and domestic workload	• Medical exam recorded neck disorders in 1969 • In 1993, 17 questions from 1969 interview used for follow-up structured medical interview to record neck, shoulders, hands and wrists disorders	• PR in 1969 and 1993 • CIR for 1970 – 1992: • Analysis adjusted for age • Cox proportional hazards models for multivariate analysis	• For neck disorders in women in 1993: ○ Overtime associated with PR of 2.3 (CI 1.0 – 5.0; age adjusted) ○ Combination of both overtime and additional domestic workload associated with PR of 3.3 (CI 1.3 – 8.6; age adjusted), with 0.6 excess risk due to the interaction • For neck disorders in men from 1970 to 1992: ○ Combination of both overtime and additional domestic workload associated with CIR of 3.0 (CI 1.1 – 8.6), with 0.6 excess risk due to the interaction • For shoulder disorders in women in 1993: ○ Overtime associated with PR of 2.7 (CI = 1.1 – 6.9; multivariate analysis)
Kawakami et al. 1999	2,194 male managers, clerks, mechanics, machine operators at one electrical plant who did not have diabetes or cardiovascular disease: • Age R 18 – 60 • Japan	Questionnaire in 1984 and 1985: • Overtime h/month: ○ < 25 h (8 – 9 h/day, 40 – 46 h/wk) ○ 26 – 50 h (9 – 10 h/day, 47 – 52 h/wk) ○ > 50 h (10+ h/day 53+ h/wk) • Schedules were day shift or rotating 2 – 3 shifts, including nights with weekly forward rotation	• Urine/blood glucose measured annually from 1984 to 1992 • Glucose tolerance test as needed • Diagnosis based on WHO criteria	• Cox's proportional hazard model • Covariates: age, education, BMI, alcohol consumption, smoking, physical activity, family history, shift work, occupation, job strain, social support at work, new technology at work	Increased risk (RR = 3.73, CI 1.4 – 9.9) associated with > 50 h overtime as compared with < 25 h while controlling for covariates
Kirkaldy et al. 2000	262 public and private managers: • Women 66% • Age R 18 – 65 • Germany	Source not clearly reported: work h/wk < 48; > 48	One-time physical symptom subscale, created from *Pressure Management Indicator*, a 120 item survey	Multiple one-way ANOVA	Physical symptoms not significant

Table 4. Studies Examining Overtime and Other Illnesses: Methods and Findings (Continued)

Author, Date	Sample	Measure of Overtime	Other Illness Measure	Statistical Methods Controls	Results Reported By Authors
Mizoue et al. 2001[a]	1,281 municipal employees: • Age not reported • Men 72% • Japan	One-time questionnaire (overtime hours during previous month 0 – < 10; 10 < 30; ≥ 30)	One-time questionnaire: • Sick building syndrome symptoms • Environmental tobacco smoke (ETS)	• Multivariate logistic regression • Covariates: age, gender, position type, asthma or hay fever, VDT use, work interest, work overload, work control, colleague support, distress, sports activity, sleep hours	• Percent of workers active in sports by overtime group: < 10h = 17%; 10 < 30h = 16%; ≥ 30 h = 8% • Percent of workers in overtime groups with ETS: < 10h = 49%; 10 < 30h = 59%; ≥ 30 h = 62% • Working overtime ≥ 30 h/month increased risk of at least one sick building syndrome symptom (OR 2.6, CI 1.4 – 4.5; adjusted for some covariates) • OR 2.96 for ≥ 30 h when adjusting for fixed covariates (age, etc) • Addition to model of lifestyle and stress-related covariates reduced OR to 2.5
Nakanishi et al. 2001a	1,266 male office workers free of impaired fasting glucose (IFG), type 2 diabetes mellitus (DM2), or history in 1994: • Age M 46, R 35 – 59 • Japan	Interview in 1994: work h/wk < 8.0; 8.0 – 8.9; 9.0 – 9.9; 10.0 – 10.9; ≥11.0	• Questionnaires and medical measurements during an annual health examination from 1994 to 1999 • American Diabetes Association guidelines used to define IFG and DM2 by fasting plasma glucose	• Cox's proportional hazards model • Covariates: age, BMI, occupation, position, smoking, alcohol, eating habits, physical activity, family history of diabetes, blood pressure, fasting glucose, total cholesterol, high density lipoprotein	• Risk of developing IFG or DM2 decreased in a dose-dependent manner with an increase in work h/day. • Reference group: < 8 h/day. • Adjusted relative risk for ≥ 11h/day was 0.50 (CI .25 – .98).
Nylén et al. 2001	20,632 workers with job titles from Swedish twin registry: • Men 54% • Sweden	Survey in 1973: • Overtime h/wk: ≤ 5, >5 • Extra work h/wk (e.g., outside normal employment): ≤ 5, >5	*Swedish Cause of Death Registry* over a 24-y period 1973 – 1996: mortality analyzed at 5 y and 24 y in the final models	• Cox's proportional hazards model: separate models for men and women • Covariates in 1973: age, marital status, smoking, alcohol use, tranquilizer use, extraversion and serious illness	• In women when controlling for other factors, > 5-h/wk overtime increased mortality at 24 y follow-up (RR = 1.92, CI 1.13 – 3.25). • In men when controlling for other factors, ≤ 5-h/wk overtime reduced mortality at 24-y follow-up (RR 0.58, CI 0.43 – 0.80), while > 5 h/wk increased mortality at 5-y follow-up (RR 2.0, CI 1.02 – 3.95), and extra work hours increased mortality at 5-y follow-up (RR 2.57, CI 1.2 – 5.52).
Siu and Donald 1995	332 workers from broad range of occupations: • Women 57% • Age R 18 – 55 • Hong Kong	One-time interview: • Overtime: yes/no • Paid for overtime: yes/no • Night or rotating: yes/no	One-time interview: Health complaints scale of 14 psychological, physical, medical symptoms	• Multiple regression • Covariates: gender, environmental conditions, and relationship with supervisor and coworkers	• Overtime associated with more health complaints (β = 0.149, p < 0.001). • Payment for overtime decreased health complaints in men (β = -0.13, p > 0.05).

Table 4. Studies Examining Overtime and Other Illnesses: Methods and Findings (Continued)

Author, Date	Sample	Measure of Overtime	Other Illness Measure	Statistical Methods Controls	Results Reported By Authors
Tuntiseranee et al. 1998	907 pregnant women and male partners who planned pregnancy and worked for pay before pregnancy: • Thailand	One-time questionnaire and clinic interview during pregnancy: • Work h/wk: <60, 61 – 70, 71 • Shift work: yes/no	• Sub-fecundity from antenatal clinic records for length of unprotected intercourse • Months to pregnancy categories tested: > 7.8; > 9.5; > 12	• Kaplan-Meier survival analysis curve • Logistic regression controlled for age, education, BMI, menstrual regularity, medical history, coital frequency, exposure to toxic agents, birth control injection, breast feeding	• Working > 71 h/wk increased risk (OR 2.3, CI 1.0 – 5.0) in primigravid and in all pregnant women (OR 1.6, CI 1.0 – 2.7) for > 9.5 months to pregnancy. • When both men and women worked > 70 h/wk, the odds ratio increased to 4.1 (CI 1.3 – 13.4) in primigravid and 2.0 (CI 1.1 – 3.8) for > 9.5 months to pregnancy for all pregnant women. • In men, work hours showed no association.
van der Hulst and Geurts 2001	535 full-time* postal workers and managers: • Age M 43.6 y • Men 95% • Netherlands *Full time = 38 h/wk*	One-time questionnaire: • Overtime h/wk dichotomized: no overtime versus ≥ 1 h/wk • Interaction 1: pressure to work overtime (low/high) and rewards (low/high) • Interaction 2: overtime (no/yes) and rewards (low/high)	One-time questionnaire dichotomized items: • Pressure to work overtime • Job and career awards • Recovery time • Burn-out • Work-home interference • "Psychomatic" health complaint scale of 13 items	• Multivariate logistic regression • Covariates: age, gender, executive position, partner status, and parental status	• Overtime with low reward associated with poor recovery, burnout, negative work-home interference (risks increased 2.2 – 3.4 times over group with no overtime high reward). "Psychosomatic" complaints NS. • Low reward with no overtime showed similar risks. • Low rewards and high pressure to work overtime was associated with adverse "psychosomatic" complaints. burnout, poor recovery, negative work-home interference (risks increased 2.6 to 8.1 times over group with no overtime and high rewards).
Voss et al. 2001	2,628 postal workers: • Men 54% • Age M men 39.5 y • Age M women 42.9 y • Sweden	One-time questionnaire asked about workplace in 1993: • > 50 h overtime (yes/no) • Other dichotomized work schedule features: full time/part time, shift work, flexible hours, desired hours	*Sweden Post's* register of absenteeism for 1993 established: • low incidence: < two events/y • high incidence: ≥ two events/y	• Multivariate logistic regression • Covariates: 150 physical, psychosocial and organizational factors tested	> 50 h overtime/y associated with lower incidence of sickness absence while controlling for other factors (men OR 0.70, CI 0.53 – 0.91; women OR 0.58, CI 0.43 – 0.79)
Worrall and Cooper 1999	1,312 managers: • Gender/age—not specified • United Kingdom	One-time questionnaire: work h/wk < 35 to > 60	One-time questionnaire: perception of health	Percent by managerial type	Report that long work hours adversely affect health: • 59% of all managers • 75% working > 60 h/wk • 21% working < 35 h/wk

Note. Abbreviations used: BMI = body mass index; BP = blood pressure; CI = 95% confidence interval; CIR = cumulative incidence ratio; D = day; E = evening; h = hours; M = mean; N = night; NS = not significant; OR = odds ratio; PR = prevalence risk ratio; R = range; RR = relative risk ratio; wk = week; y = years.
[a] Mizoue reference appears also in Table 6.

3.1c Overtime and Injuries

Table 5 displays the methods and results for the studies examining overtime and injuries. Two studies reported that overtime was associated with higher on-the-job injury rates in construction workers or health care workers [Lowery et al. 1998; Simpson and Severson 2000]. Åkerstedt et al. [2002], however, reported no relationship between more than 50 hours of work per week and work-related fatalities in a 20-year prospective Swedish study.

3.1d Overtime and Health Behaviors

Table 6 displays the methods and results for the studies examining overtime and health behaviors. Studies by Nakamura et al. [1998] and Shields [1999] reported that overtime was associated with increased odds for unhealthy weight gain in men. Shields also reported that changing from a 40-hour workweek to longer working hours raised the odds for smoking in both men and women. In contrast, Park et al. [2001b] found no difference in smoking across three groups of engineers whose work hours ranged from a minimum of 52 hours per week to a maximum of 89 hours.

Differences in alcohol consumption also varied among studies. Shields [1999] reported a U-shaped relationship: women who either reduced or increased their average hours worked per week during the previous two years increased their odds for higher alcohol consumption. Trinkoff and Storr [1998] reported higher alcohol consumption in nurses was associated with working more overtime shifts per month. Park et al. [2001b] reported no differences in alcohol use among engineers whose work hours ranged from minimum of 52 hours per week to a maximum of 89 hours.

Mizoue et al. [2001] found a significant decrease in the percentage of workers who participated in regular sports activity as overtime hours increased. Studies by Shields [1999] and Kageyama et al. [1998], however, reported no significant relationship between long working hours and leisure-time physical activity.

3.1e Overtime and Performance

Table 6 displays the methods and results for the studies examining overtime and performance. Proctor et al. [1996] investigated 248 United Auto Workers working day and evening shifts. The researchers reported poorer performance on tests of cognitive function (e.g., Trail-making Test, Wisconsin Card Sort Task, Symbol Digit Substitution Task, Visual Reproduction, Pattern Memory, Vocabulary Task) and executive function (the ability to prioritize and plan tasks) for those individuals who worked overtime as compared with those who did not. Kirkcaldy et al. [1997] reported that as work hours increased in health care workers, automobile crashes and on the job "accidents" increased.

3.2 FINDINGS ASSOCIATED WITH EXTENDED WORK SHIFTS

Twelve field studies and three laboratory studies examined associations between extended work shifts and the outcomes targeted for this report. The field studies were conducted in United States (4), Australia (2), Sweden (2), United Kingdom (2), France (1), and Germany (1). The studies compared a variety of extended shift schedules: 12-hour day shifts and 12-hour night shifts; 8-hour rotations and 12-hour rotations; 8-hour and 10-hour rotations. Injuries and performance across the 1st hour through the 12th hour of long shifts were also examined. Table 7 displays the methods and results for studies that examined extended work shifts.

Table 5. Studies Examining Overtime and Injuries: Methods and Findings

Author, Date	Sample	Measure of Overtime	Health or Safety Measure	Statistical Methods Controls	Results Reported By Authors
Åkerstedt et al. 2002	47,680 employed men and women beginning at age 16 (total cohort): • Sweden	Interviewed regularly for 20 y: work h/wk < 50 or > 50	Occupational fatality from *Swedish Cause of Death Registry* across 20 y	• Cox regression survival analysis • Covariates: demographics, sleep, other work characteristics	No significant relationship reported between >50 h/wk and occupational fatality.
Lowery et al. 1998	2,140 airport construction contracts involving approximately 32,000 workers (men 95%): • Employed 12/1990 to 8/1994. • Age R 15 – 60⁺ • United States	Percent of payroll that was overtime by contract: 0%, >0% – 20%, >20%	4,634 paid workers' compensation claims to determine: • Non-lost work time (non-LWT) injury rate • Lost work time (LWT) injury rate	Poisson regression	• Numbers of LWT injuries were small and NS. • Rate ratio for non-LWT injuries increased to 1.57 (CI 1.13 – 2.17) for contracts with > 20% overtime.
Simpson and Severson 2000	2,247 workers from one hospital: • 155 injured and 2,092 non-injured • Age not reported • Women 81% • United States	From 1997 hospital records: hours worked < 2000; ≥ 2000	Hospital injury records in 1997: cut, fracture, sprain, amputation, etc.	• Logistic regression • Covariates: age, gender, ethnicity, job title, physical demand rating, work hours obtained from hospital records	Working ≥ 2000 h/y increased risk for injury (OR 1.71, CI = 1.22 – 2.38).

Note. Abbreviations used: BMI = body mass index; BP = blood pressure; CI = 95% confidence interval; CIR = cumulative incidence ratio; D = day; E = evening; h = hours; M = mean; N = night; NS = not significant; OR = odds ratio; PR = prevalence risk ratio; R = range; RR = relative risk ratio; wk = week; y = years

Table 6. Studies Examining Overtime Health Behaviors, and Performance Outcomes: Methods and Findings

Author, Date	Sample	Measure of Overtime	Health or Safety Measure	Statistical Methods Controls	Results Reported By Authors
Kageyama et al. 1998	223 male *white collar* workers: • Age M 30.8 • Japan	One-time questionnaire and interview (overtime h/month < 20; 20 – 59; >60)	One-time questionnaire and interview measured exercise: rarely, 1 – 2/month, 1 wk, ≥ 2/wk	• General linear models • Covariates: age, body mass index, smoking and alcohol intake, commute time • Kendall's rank correlation	Frequency of exercise not correlated with overtime
Kirkcaldy et al. 1997	2,500 health care workers: • Women 87% • Age M 33, R 15 – 86 • Germany	One-time questionnaire: work h/wk	One-time questionnaire: driving crashes and job-related "accidents"	• Multiple regression • Covariates: age, gender, work climate, commute distance, job stress, children	As work hours increased, job-related "accidents" and driving crashes increased (p < 05)
Mizoue et al. 2001[a]	1,281 municipal employees: • Age not reported • Men 72% • Japan	One-time questionnaire (overtime hours during previous month 0 – < 10; 10 < 30; ≥ 30)	One-time questionnaire: • Sick building syndrome symptoms • Environmental tobacco smoke (ETS)	• Multivariate logistic regression • Covariates: age, gender, position type, asthma or hay fever, VDT use, work interest, work overload, work control, colleague support, distress, sports activity, sleep hours	• Percent of workers active in sports by overtime group: < 10h = 17%; 10 < 30h = 16%; ≥ 30 h = 8% • Percent of workers in overtime groups with ETS: < 10h = 49%; 10 < 30h = 59%; ≥ 30 h = 62% • Working overtime ≥ 30 h/month increased risk of at least one sick building syndrome symptom (OR 2.6, CI 1.4 – 4.5; adjusted for some covariates) • OR 2.96 for ≥ 30 h when adjusting for fixed covariates (age, etc) • Addition to model of lifestyle and stress-related covariates reduced OR to 2.5
Nakamura et al. 1998	248 male non-management *white collar* workers: • Age M 31, R 21 – 56 • Japan	• From time clocks between 1990 and 1993 • Overtime: average monthly work hours beyond 40 h/wk	1990 and 1993 measured height, weight, abdominal and hip circumference, skin-fold thickness, serum cholesterol/triglycerides.	• Pearson, Spearman Correlation • Multiple linear regression with stepwise procedures • Covariates: age, gender, marital status, education and lifestyle (e.g., eating habits, exercise, smoking, alcohol use)	• Increased overtime correlated with an increase in BMI (r = .172, p < .01) and waist circumference (r = .218, p<0.01) from 1990 to 1993, but not with 1993 measurements alone. • While controlling for late dinner, overtime associated with an increase in BMI (ß = 0.0103, p < 0.05). • While controlling for age, overtime associated with an increase in waist circumference (ß= 0.0405, p < 0.05).
Park et al. 2001b	238 male engineers from 3 electronics manufacturing plants: • Age M 32 • South Korea	One-time questionnaire (M h/wk during previous month):* < 60; > 60 < 70; > 70 * R 52 – 89 h/wk	One-time questionnaire: • Number of cigarettes per day • Number of alcoholic drinks per week	• Analysis of covariance adjusting for age • Duncan's multiple comparison procedure	No significant differences in mean number of daily cigarettes smoked or mean number of weekly alcohol drinks across the three working hour groups

Table 6. Studies Examining Overtime, Health Behaviors, and Perfomance Outcomes: Methods and Findings (Continued)

Author, Date	Sample	Measure of Overtime	Health or Safety Measure	Statistical Methods Controls	Results Reported By Authors

Proctor et al. 1996	248 hourly paid automotive workers:
	• Age M 36
	• Men 64%
	• United States
		Overtime calculated from payroll records week before test day:
		• Overtime defined as hours > 8 per shift or > 5 days per week
		• Shifts were fixed days or evenings
			One-time neuro-psychological test battery:
			Trail-making Test, Wisconsin Card Sort Task, Symbol-digit, Visual Reproduction, Recognition Test, Pattern Memory, Vocabulary Test
				• Pearson's correlation
				• Student's t-test
				• Multiple linear stepwise regression models
				• Covariates: age, education, gender, alcohol use, repeated school grade, petroleum naphtha exposure, shift, job type, number consecutive days worked before testing, and number work hours on test day
					• Mean test performance for overtime group tended to be worse than comparison group for 15 of 24 tasks (primarily areas of attention and executive function).
					• Three reached statistical significance:
					  ○ Time to complete Trails B (β = 1.6, CI 0.66 – 2.5)
					  ○ 2-min recall on Delayed Recognition Span Test
					  ○ The Vocabulary Test (Student's t test, p < 0.05)
					• In final models, overtime predicted impaired performance on Trails A, Trails B, Wisconsin Card Sorting, and Vocabulary tests.

Sheilds 1999	• Randomly selected sample of 2.181 men, 1.649 women in the *National Population Health Survey* from various occupations:
	• Work ≥ 35 h/week entire year before 1994/1995
	• Age R 25 – 54
	• Canada
		Phone interviews in 1994/95 and 1996/97:
		• Work h/wk: 35 – 40 (standard); ≥ 41 (long).
		• Shift type: day versus all types of shift work.
			Phone interviews in 1994/95 and 1996/97:
			• Alcohol: number of drinks/day during week before interview
			• Smoking: number of cigarettes/day
			• Weight: BMI, underweight BMI < 20; acceptable BMI, 20 – 24.9; some excess BMI, 25 – 27; overweight BMI > 27.
			• Physical activity: number of times ≥ 15 minutes during last 3 months
				• Multiple logistic regression models run separately for men and women
				• Covariates: age, marital status, household income, presence of children < 12 at home, education, stress occupation, shift work, self-employment, multiple jobs, high job strain, job insecurity, low supervisor support
					• Alcohol consumption:
					  ○ Women who either increased (standard to long hours) or reduced hours (long hours to standard) showed increased risk (2.0, CI: 1.1 – 3.4; 1.6, CI: 1.0 – 2.6 respectively) for higher alcohol consumption
					  ○ Men who increased weekly hours were not associated with more alcohol consumption, and reduction in their work hours decreased odds of increasing consumption (0.5, CI: 0.3 – 0.9)
					• BMI:
					  ○ Men who moved from standard hours to long hours showed increase odds (2.2, CI: 1.2 – 4.0) for weight gain compared to men who continued to work standard hours
					  ○ Men who worked long hours increased odds for excess weight by 1.4
					  ○ No significant changes for women
					• Smoking:
					  ○ Men who changed from standard to long working hours increased the odds (2.2, CI: 1.1 – 4.5) of smoking more
					  ○ Women increased their odds even more (4.1, CI: 1.4 – 11.6)
					• Exercise showed no significant changes.

Table 6. Studies Examining Overtime, Health Behaviors, and Performance Outcomes: Methods and Findings (Continued)

Author, Date	Sample	Measure of Overtime	Health or Safety Measure	Statistical Methods Controls	Results Reported By Authors

Trinkoff and Storr 1998[b]	National random sample of 3,917 registered nurses employed full- or part-time:
	• Age M 43
	• 95% women
	• United States
		One-time questionnaire:
		• Number h/day: > 8; ≤ 8
		• Overtime days/month 0, 1 – 3, 4 – 7, ≥ 8
		• Shift type: day, evening, night
		• Rotation: yes/no
		• Interaction: shift by hours worked/day
			One-time questionnaire:
			• Drug use in past year yes/no: marijuana, cocaine, prescription drug use without prescription
			• Alcohol use: 5 or more drinks on one occasion
			• Smoking: > 10 cigarettes /day
				Logistic regression adjusted for demographics	• Overtime and shift length NS for drug use.
					• Risk for smoking increased with > 8-h night shifts (OR 1.62; CI 1.14 – 2.31).
					• Risk for alcohol increased:
					  ○ > 8-h (OR 1.44; CI 1.2 – 1.72) versus ≤ 8-h
					  ○ 1 to 7 days overtime/month (OR 1.44 – 1.49)
					  ○ > 8-h night (OR 1.4; CI 1 – 1.98) and > 8-h rotating shifts (OR 1.52; CI 1.04 – 2.22)

Note. Abbreviations used: β = beta; BMI = body mass index; BP = blood pressure; CI = 95% confidence interval; CIR = cumulative incidence ratio; D = day; E = evening; h = hours; M = mean; N = night; NS = not significant; OR = odds ratio; PR = prevalence risk ratio; R = range; RR = relative risk ratio; wk = week; y = years.
[a] Mizoue reference appears also in Table 4. [b] Trinkoff and Storr reference appears also in Table 7.

16

3.2a Extended Work Shifts and Illnesses

Lipscomb et al. [2002] reported that working 12 or more hours per shift was associated with increased risk for back disorders in nurses when compared with an 8-hour shift. Prunier-Poulmaire et al. [1998] reported that a 12-hour fast rotation (shift change more than once a week) was associated with increased leg pain, and visual complaints, as compared with day shift. In addition, the 8-hour 3-shift rotation showed increased risk for more leg pain, as well as more cardiovascular and gastrointestinal complaints, when compared with day shift. In contrast, Johnson and Sharit [2001] reported that a 12-hour fast rotation was associated with better perceived general health and fewer gastrointestinal complaints when compared with a fast 8-hour 3-shift rotation.

Smith et al. [1998] compared 12-hour day-night rotations with flexible start times and 12-hour rotations with rigid start times, but found no differences in cardiovascular, gastrointestinal, or pain symptoms.

3.2b Extended Work Shifts and Injuries

Hänecke et al. [1998] analyzed 1.2 million injury reports from two national databases in Germany and reported a higher risk for injury after the 8th or 9th hour at work for all shifts. The report indicated more pronounced risk for evening and night shifts as compared to days. Macias et al. [1996] examined hospital incident reports for a 30-month period at one university hospital in the United States and reported that needlestick and biological fluid exposure rates increased during the last 2 hours of 12-hour shifts, whereas no increase occurred during the last 2 hours of 8-hour shifts. Johnson and Sharit [2001], however, reported that production workers who changed from an 8-hour to a 12-hour shift did not show an increase in recordable injuries or lost-time incidents after the change.

3.2c Extended Work Shifts and Health Behaviors

Trinkoff and Storr [1998] reported increased odds for higher alcohol use in nurses who worked longer rotating or night shifts and increased odds for smoking in nurses who worked extended night shifts. No relationship was reported between working hours and drug abuse.

3.2d Extended Work Shifts and Performance

Two laboratory studies reported deterioration in performance with extended shifts. Rosa et al. [1998] compared a 2-week 12-hour day/night rotation and a 2-week 8-hour day-night rotation using a simulated manual assembly task at three repetition rates and three torque loads. They reported that upper extremity fatigue increased more quickly with increasing time on shift and occurred more quickly during night shifts. The highest fatigue levels were found during 12-hour night shifts. Macdonald and Bendak [2000] compared a 12-hour shift to a more standard workday (7.2 hours) in a laboratory study and reported that the longer workday was associated with deterioration in grammatical reasoning and alertness.

In contrast, four field studies reported no differences in their performance measures during extended shifts. Schroeder et al. [1998] reported that air traffic control personnel working four 10-hour shifts did not significantly differ from personnel working five 8-hour shifts on tests of grammatical reasoning, reaction time, and digit addition although performance of both groups declined across the workweek. Similarly, Smith et al. [1995] reported no significant declines in alertness or cognitive performance between 8-hour and 12-hour shifts in nuclear power plant shift workers. Axelsson et al. [1998] reported no significant difference in simple reaction time and vigilance task measures between 8- and 12-hour shifts in Swedish power plant workers. Also, Lowden et al. [1998] reported no consistent

Table 7. Studies Examining Extended Work Shifts: Methods and Findings

Author, Date	Sample	Description of Work Schedule	Health or Safety Measure	Statistical Methods Controls	Results Reported By Authors
Axelsson et al. 1998	28 power plant workers: • Gender/age not clearly reported for performance testing • Sweden	3-shift fast forward rotation with 8-h shifts Monday to Thursday, 12-h shifts Friday to Sunday (4 – 7 on, 2 – 10 off). M 35 h/wk	Simple reaction time and 10 minute vigilance tests compared 8-h and 12-h shifts at the beginning and end of 3 day shifts and 3 night shifts	Repeated measures ANOVA with Huynh-Feldt epsilon correction method	No significant performance differences between 8-h and 12-h shifts on simple reaction time tests and vigilance tasks.
Brake and Bates 2001	• 45 male underground miners acclimatized to hot work environment • 15 controls in sedentary thermoneutral conditions • Australia	• First summer worked 6-h shifts • Intervention during next summer was self-paced 10-h, 12-h, or 12.5-h shifts • Data collected during day and night shifts, but did not report time-of-day effects • Work h/wk not reported	Pre- and post-intervention at shift start, middle, and end for several shifts collected continuous heart rate: • Polar ECG-type recorders • Cycle ergometer heart rates with pedal rate = 50 rpm at 100 Watts	Student's t-test	• No significant changes in full shift continuous heart rate reported between 6-h shifts and self-paced extended shifts. • Cycle ergometer heart rate showed significant increase between start and end of shift ($p<.01$). • In 24 workers measured at start, middle, and end of extended shifts, ergometer heart rate showed significant increase between shift start and mid-shift ($P=0.001$), followed by significant decrease between mid-shift and shift end ($p=0.04$).
Hanecke et al. 1998	1.2 million workers' compensation records for "accidents" at work: • Gender/age not reported • Germany	1994 Workers' compensation records: • Hour at work when "accident" occurred: 1st to 12th hour, > 12th hour • Time of day "accident" occurred • Interaction: time of day by hour at work	• 1994 workers' compensation records of "accident" at work leading to > 3 days absence • Used two German work hour surveys in 1992 and 1993 to estimate population exposed (the denominator)	• Chi Square • Relative risk	• Relative risk for "accident" increased exponentially beyond the 9th hour at work. • Interaction for time of day by hour at work ((Chi-square = 71484, df = 264; $p < 0.0001$) suggests "accident" risk beyond 8th or 9th hour was greater for evening and night shifts as compared with days.
Johnson and Sharit 2001	Production workers at one manufacturing site: • One division (n = 350, 90% male) that changed shift length was compared with other divisions (n = about 7700, 84% male) • Age groups: > 30, 30 – 39, 40 – 49, >50 • United States	• 8-h 3-shift rotation changed to 12-h day/night rotation • Work h/wk not available	• OSHA work-related injury/illness records examined over 10 years (2 y before schedule change, 8 y after change) • *Hours of Work Questionnaire* measured overall health and digestive symptoms while on 8-h shifts, 11 months after change to 12-h shifts, and 8 y after change	• Z-scores adjusted for age and gender • Tested standardized incident/illness rate, lost time case rate, lost workday rate • Chi Square for independence tested digestive symptoms	• Significant increases found only in control group for injury rates, lost time case rates, lost workday rates (all $p <.05$). • Digestive symptoms and overall perceived health showed improvement after changing to 12-h schedule ($p < 0.001$).
Lipscomb et al. 2002[a]	1,163 working nurses randomly selected from two states: • Age M 45 • Women 95% • United States	One-time questionnaire: • Work h/day: ≤ 8; 9 – 11; ≥12 • Work h/wk: ≤40; 41 – 49; ≥50 • Work days/wk: 1 – 5; 6 – 7 • Day shift versus other • Interactions: h/shift by h/wk	One-time *Nordic Survey of Musculoskeletal Symptoms*	Logistic regression adjusted for age	• Compared to 8-h shift, ≥ 12-h/day increased risk for back disorders (OR 1.61, CI 1.05 – 2.48). • Interactions suggested that ≥ 12-h/day combined with ≥ 40-h/week elevated risk for disorders of neck (OR 2.30, CI 1.03 – 5.11), shoulder (OR 2.48, CI 1.07 – 5.77), and back (OR 2.67, CI 1.26 – 5.66).
Lowden et al. 1998	14 shift workers, 9 day workers at a chemical plant: • Gender/age not reported for subsample • Sweden	8-h 3-shift backward fast rotation with M 40 h/wk changed to 12-h day/night fast rotation (2N, 5 off, 2D, 2 off, 3N) with M 36 h/wk	Before shift change and 10 months after tested simple visual reaction time at beginning and end of shift	• ANOVA • Chi square • Newman-Keuls post hoc procedures	Simple visual reaction-time results showed no differences in performance with the change from an 8-h 3-shift rotation to a 12-h day/night rotation.

Table 7. Studies Examining Extended Work Shifts: Methods and Findings (Continued)

Author, Date	Sample	Description of Work Schedule	Health or Safety Measure	Statistical Methods Controls	Results Reported By Authors
Macdonald and Bendak 2000	• Two laboratory studies: ○ 2 men and 2 women performing cognitive tasks; ○ 2 men and 2 women performing high physical work ○ age M 29.5 • Field study ○ production operators at one plant: 12-h shift n = 17 men; 8-h shift n = 17; 76% male ○ Age R 21 – 61 • Australia	• Laboratory study: ○ High physical work lab study compared 7.2-h 5-day week with 12-h 3-day week ○ Cognitive task lab study compared 7.2-h days during 1 wk at low workload, 1 wk at high workload, and 12-h days during 1 wk at high workload, 1 wk at low workload • Field study: ○ Plant schedules: 8-h fixed day or day/evening weekly rotation; 12-h day/night biweekly rotation (2 –3 on, 2 – 3 off): h/wk not reported ○ Interactions: workday duration and workload	• Lab study assessment battery items: bodily discomfort chart with rating scales, alertness ratings, workload ratings, hand steadiness, Critical Flicker Fusion, Grammatical Reasoning, dual task (Grammatical Reasoning and auditory choice reaction time), simultaneous pattern comparison, tapping • Field study measures: job analysis, workload measurement, personal characteristics questionnaire, assessment battery at start, middle, end of 3 day shifts	• Repeated measures ANOVA • Regression analysis • Other factors in the analysis: demographics, health, commute time, job coping skills, alertness rating, bodily discomfort score	• In laboratory study, 12-h shift showed decreased self-rated alertness ($F=10.65$, $p < 0.05$), increased grammatical reasoning errors ($F=11.83$, $p < 0.05$), higher perceived physical workload ratings ($F=10.14$, $p <0.05$). 12-h shifts with high cognitive tasks showed slightly more errors than 7.2-h shifts while 12-h shifts with low cognitive tasks showed marginally better performance. • In field study, increases in workloads on 12-h shifts showed increased discomfort and grammatical reasoning errors, and deterioration in alertness and hand steadiness.
Macias et al. 1996	• 393 biological hazard exposure incidents to health care workers in one hospital: • Age gender not reported • United States	Retrospective record review of work schedule data over 30 months: • Hour into workday when incident occurred • 8-h shift versus 12-h (> 12-h shifts excluded)	• Biological hazardous exposure obtained from hospital records over 30 months • Number of workers exposed, number of hazardous procedures obtained from records or estimated	• Kolmogorov-Smirnov one sample test • ANOVA with Tukey procedure	• Exposures per worker increased last 2 hours of 12-h shift ($F = 5.75$, $p < 0.01$). • Exposures per procedure increased risk during first hour into shift ($F=5.62$, $p <0.01$) and last 2 hours of 12-h shift ($F=5.75$, $p<0.01$). • No increased risk during last hours of 8-h shift.
Prunier-Poulmaire et al. 1998	• 302 customs service workers from 44 national units: • Age/gender distribution not clearly reported • France	• Types of schedules: ○ Day shift reference group ○ 6-h 4-shift fast rotation ○ 8-h 3-shift fast rotation ○ 12-h day/night fast rotation • Work h/wk not specified	One-time questionnaire measured gastrointestinal and cardiovascular complaints, medications, eating habits, caffeine and smoking consumption, sleep difficulties.	• Logistic regression • Covariates: age, gender, physically demanding job, boring job, conflicts with travelers	• 12-h day/night rotation was associated with visual problems (OR 3.0, CI 1.14 – 7.77), and pain in the legs (OR 3.4, CI 1.36 – 8.26) compared with the day shift reference group. • 8-h 3-shift rotation and 6-h 4-shift rotation had 3-fold or more increase in cardiovascular, gastrointestinal, sleeping, and leg complaints compared with the day-shift reference group.
Reid and Dawson 2001	• 32 participants in laboratory study divided into two age groups: • Younger group of 4 women and 12 men, M age 21, R 18 – 30 • Older group of 3 women and 13 men, M age 44, R 35 – 56; • Australia	Simulated 12-h shift schedule: • DDNN • Interaction: age by shift	Every hour carried out three 1-minute compensatory tracking tests of the *Occupational Safety Performance Assessment Test* (OPSAT).	• Repeated measures ANOVA • Bonferroni tests • Simple regression analyses	• Performance consistently lower in older workers, including baseline ($p <$ .002) and each shift (Day shift 1, $p <$ .0001; Day shift 2, $p <$ .0001; Night shift 1, $p <$ .0001; Night shift 2, $p <$ .0001). • Performance significantly increased across day shifts and decreased across nights in the older group, but remained stable in the younger group.
Rosa et al. 1998	• 16 participants in laboratory study assigned randomly to one of four simulated shift schedules: • 50% male • Age R 21 – 40 • United States	• Simulated shift schedules: ○ 8-h: 5D, 2 off, 5N ○ 8-h: 5N, 2 off, 5D ○ 12-h: 4D, 3 off, 4N ○ 12-h: 4N, 3 off, 4D • Interaction: shift length by shift time of day (day versus night)	Simulated manual assembly work tasks that manipulated load and repetition rates: • Upper extremity fatigue using the Borg CR-10 scale • *Yoshitake Questionnaire for Subjective Symptoms of Fatigue*	Repeated measures ANOVA: 2 schedules (8-h versus 12-h) X 4 days X 2 shifts (day versus night) X 3 load levels X 3 repetition rates	• Highest fatigue observed during 12-h night shifts. Similar fatigue levels reached at end of both weeks of 8-h night shifts and 12-h day shifts. • Fatigue observed more quickly with increasing time on shifts and with night shifts compared with day shifts.

Table 7. Studies Examining Extended Work Shifts: Methods and Findings (Continued)

Author, Date	Sample	Description of Work Schedule	Health or Safety Measure	Statistical Methods Controls	Results Reported By Authors
Schroeder et al. 1998[b]	52 air traffic controllers: • Age M 37.9, R 28 – 50 • Men 86% • United States	Compared 8-h fast backward rotation (EEDDN) and 10-h fast rotation (EEDD)	Cognitive performance using the NIOSH fatigue test battery (choice reaction time, digit addition, grammatical reasoning), administered three times each workday for 3 weeks.	• Least squares regression • Repeated measures ANOVA • Newman-Keuls tests to determine significant mean differences across day of work week and test session	• Test battery performance on the 10-h rotation no different from 8-h rotation when the initial 4 days of the work week were compared • Poorer performance for night shift • For both schedules, decrements were observed on some of the NIOSH performance measures at the end of the workday and at the end of the workweek.

Smith et al. 1995	22 male nuclear power plant workers:
	• Divided into two groups:
	  ○ 11 engineer + reactor operators (EROP)
	  ○ 11 craftsmen + maintenance (CMOP)
	• Age M 42
	• United Kingdom
		• Both groups worked 8-h 3-shift backward rotation, but the EROP group also worked two 12-h day shifts and two 12-h night shifts in their 35-day cycle
		• Work h/wk not specified
			Obtained every 2 hours during 8 selected shifts:
			• Computerized test battery (choice reaction time, memory search task [SAM-5])
			• 20 pt. visual analog scale to subjectively assess alertness
				• Repeated measures ANOVA and Turkey's tests used for post hoc comparisons
				• Two types of analysis for entire group: outcome measures x shift type (e.g., day, evening, night) and outcome measures x 2-h time intervals during work shift
					• No significant difference between 8-h and 12-h shifts on alertness or cognitive performance
					• No major group by shift type or time on shift interaction effects were found.

Smith et al. 1998	92 police officers at four sites:
	• Age M 42.4
	• Gender not reported
	• United Kingdom
		• Two control sites on 8-h 3-shift fast backward rotation, M 42 h/wk, n= 44
		• Two trial sites on 8-h rotation changed to 12-h day/night fast forward rotation (2D, 2N, 3 off), M 39 h/wk, n = 48
		  ○ Flexible start times at one site
		  ○ Rigid 6 a.m. start time at other site
			Data collection pre- and 6 months post-work schedule change at all four sites: alertness and physical symptoms in *Standard Shiftwork Index*.	• ANOVA
				• ANCOVA
				• Covariates: demographics, work and shift work experience, workload, job pacing, morningness, sleep flexibility, chronic fatigue
					• 12-h day shift with flexible start time showed improvements in alertness versus rigid start time.
					• Cardiovascular, gastrointestinal, pain symptoms NS.
					• Differences in shift work experience between control and trial sites prevented comparison of 8-h and 12-h shifts.

Trinkoff and Storr 1998[b]	National random sample of 3,917 registered nurses employed full- or part-time:
	• Age M 43
	• 95% women
	• United States
		One-time questionnaire:
		• Number h/day: > 8; ≤ 8
		• Overtime days/month 0, 1 – 3, 4 – 7, ≥ 8
		• Shift type: day, evening, night
		• Rotation: yes/no
		• Interaction: shift by hours worked/day
			One-time questionnaire:
			• Drug use in past year yes/no: marijuana, cocaine, prescription drug use without prescription
			• Alcohol use: 5 or more drinks on one occasion
			• Smoking: > 10 cigarettes /day
				Logistic regression adjusted for demographics	• Overtime and shift length NS for drug use
					• Risk for smoking increased with > 8-h night shifts (OR 1.62; CI 1.14 – 2.31).
					• Risk for alcohol increased:
					  ○ > 8-h (OR 1.44; CI 1.2 – 1.72) versus ≤ 8-h
					  ○ 1 to 7 days overtime/month (OR 1.44 – 1.49)
					  ○ > 8-h night (OR 1.4: CI 1 – 1.98) and > 8-h rotating shifts (OR 1.52: CI 1.04 – 2.22)

Note. Abbreviations used: BMI = body mass index; BP = blood pressure; CI = 95% confidence interval; CIR = cumulative incidence ratio; D = day; E = evening; h = hours; M = mean; N = night; NS = not significant; OR = odds ratio; OSHA = Occupational Safety and Health Administration; PR = prevalence risk ratio; R = range; RR = relative risk ratio; wk = week; y = years. [a]Lipscomb reference appears also in Table 6. [b]Trinkoff Storr reference appears also in Table 8.

differences on simple performance measures, such as reaction time, in shift workers who switched from an 8-hour to a 12-hour schedule.

The way other features of work schedules, work tasks, and work environment influenced the relationship of shift length and performance were examined by three studies. Smith et al. [1998] reported improvements in alertness in 12-hour day/night rotations with flexible start times when compared with 12-hour rotations with rigid start times. The field study by Macdonald and Bendak [2000] reported that a combination of high workload and 12-hour shifts was associated more consistently with increased errors on grammatical reasoning, greater deterioration in hand steadiness and alertness, and more discomfort when compared to high workload during 8-hour shifts.

Brake and Bates [2001] examined extended shifts in combination with heat stress in Australian underground miners. Cardiovascular fatigue assessed by continuous heart rate monitoring showed no difference between 6-hour shifts and self-paced extended shifts (10-hour to 12.5-hour shifts). Additional heart rate monitoring while riding cycle ergometers showed increases during the first half of long shifts, but decreases during the second half of the shift. Based on these results, the authors suggested that the miners had reduced their effort and were pacing themselves in the latter part of the extended shifts.

One study examined the influence of age. Reid and Dawson [2001] conducted a laboratory study of simulated 12-hour shifts and neurobehavioral performance in younger and older participants. Older laboratory subjects were less able than younger subjects to maintain performance across 12-hour shifts.

3.3 FINDINGS ASSOCIATED WITH EXTENDED WORK SHIFTS, COMBINED WITH MORE THAN 40-HOURS WORK PER WEEK

Six field studies examined extended work shifts which also had more than 40-hours of work per week. The studies in this section clearly reported that participants worked on average more than 40 hours per week over the course of several weeks. The studies were conducted in the United States (2), Australia (1), Brazil (1), Canada (1), and United Kingdom (1). A variety of 8-hour and 12-hour schedules were compared across the studies. Table 8 shows the methods and results for studies that examined extended work shifts when combined with more than 40 hours per week.

3.3a Extended Work Shifts Combined with More than 40-Hours Work per Week and Illnesses

Lipscomb et al. [2002] reported that the combination of 12-hour shifts and 40 or more hours of work a week was associated with elevated risk for neck, shoulder, and back disorders as compared to five 8-hour shifts per week. In contrast, Mitchell and Williamson [2000] reported *fewer* health complaints during a 12-hour day/night fast forward rotation when compared with an 8-hour 3-shift weekly backward rotation.

Tucker et al. [1998a] examined early and late start times in workers on 12-hour shift rotations and 8-hour 3-shift rotations. Both work schedules changed shifts more than once a week. The 12-hour shift was associated with more cardiovascular and musculoskeletal complaints than the 8-hour shift. Workers on 12-hour shifts, having early changeover time, reported the most cardiovascular and musculoskeletal complaints.

Table 8. Studies Examining Extended Work Shifts Combined with More than 40 Hours per Week: Methods and Findings

Author, Date	Sample	Description of Work Schedule	Health or Safety Measure	Statistical Methods Controls	Results Reported By Authors
Duchon et al. 1997	30 underground male miners: • Age not reported • Canada	• 8-h 3-shift rotation with M 41 h/wk changed to experimental 12-h day/night rotation (4 on, 4 off) with M 48 h/wk • Control group: 8-h day shift, 40 h/wk	• Tested pre-, mid-, post-shift for a week: ○ 8-h rotation ○ After 12-h rotation for 10 months • Submaximal exercise testing • Continuous heart rate monitoring • Computerized test battery tested pursuit tracking, grammatical reasoning, choice reaction time, finger tapping	• Three-way mixed design ANOVA • Kruskal-Wallis one-way ANOVA	• No significant main effects between 8- and 12-h shifts on neurobehavioral performance measures. • Continuous heart rate findings showed pacing of work effort on 12-h shifts relative to 8-h shifts. The 12-h workers appeared to pace their work at a slower rate than the 8-h workers.
Fischer et al. 2000	22 male workers at a petrochemical plant: • Age M 32.6; • Brazil	• 12-h day/night rapid rotation (2 – 3D, 2 – 3 N, 4 – 5 off) • 48 M h/wk	For 30 days, recorded subjective alertness at 2nd, 6th, 10th hour of day and night shifts using visual analog scale (10cm) from *not at all alert* to *very alert*.	• Repeated measures ANOVA • Tukey tests for post hoc comparisons	Significant reduction in alertness (p < 0.001): • Days, from 2nd hour to 10th hour. • Nights, 10th hour reduced from 2nd and 6th hour. • No reduction seen across successive night shifts.
Lipscomb et al. 2002[a]	1,163 working nurses randomly selected from two states: • Age M 45 • Women 95% • United States	One-time questionnaire: • Work h/day: ≤ 8; 9 – 11; ≥12 • Work h/wk: ≤40; 41 – 49; ≥50 • Work days/wk: 1 – 5; 6 – 7 • Day shift versus other • Interactions: h shift by h/wk	One-time *Nordic Survey of Musculoskeletal Symptoms*	Logistic regression adjusted for age	• Compared to 8-h shift, ≥ 12-h/day increased risk for back disorders (OR 1.61, CI 1.05 – 2.48). • Interactions suggested that ≥ 12-h/day combined with ≥ 40-h/week elevated risk for disorders of neck (OR 2.30, CI 1.03 – 5.11), shoulder (OR 2.48,CI 1.07 – 5.77), and back (OR 2.67,CI 1.26 – 5.60).

Table 8. Studies Examining Extended Work Shifts Combined with More than 40 Hours per Week: Methods and Findings (Continued)

Author, Date	Sample	Description of Work Schedule	Health or Safety Measure	Statistical Methods Controls	Results Reported By Authors
Mitchell and Williamson 2000	27 male electrical power station employees: • Age M 44 • Australia	8-h 3-shift backward weekly rotation with M 40-h/wk changed to 12-h fast forward rotation (4 on, 3 off, 5 on, 7 off, 5 on, 2 off) with M 42 h/wk	• Data collected before and 10 months after schedule change: sick leave records, workplace accident records • *Standard Shiftwork Index* to measure physical health, well-being, alcohol use • *Information and Performance Test System* for neurobehavioral performance	Multivariate ANOVA and Bonferroni correction methods with post-hoc comparisons	• More health complaints during 8-h rotation than 12-h rotation. • Alcohol/cigarette use: ○ 47% on 8-h rotation reported using alcohol as a sleep aid between night shifts compared to 17% on 12-h rotation ○ 40% on 8-h rotation smoked versus 25% on 12-h • Two "accidents" occurred during the 8-h rotation and one during the 12-h (not statistically analyzed). • On vigilance test 12-h workers made more errors on infrequent stimuli (t = -2.43, p < 0.02) at the end of both day and night shifts. • Significant improvements observed for simple reaction time and grammatical reasoning test at the end of the 12-h shift compared with the beginning. • No increase in vigilance task errors was found for the 8-h shift, but similar improvements reported at end of shift compared with beginning. • No differences reported for the critical tracking task.
Novak and Auvil-Novack 1996	45 intensive care unit nurses from 1 hospital • 96% women • Age M 34.4 • United States	• Focus groups during 1 night shift worked 48 h/wk: (four 10-h shifts/wk) • Type of schedule: 12-h fixed night or 12-h day/night rotation	Focus groups during 1 night shift discussed automobile crash or near miss and job performance	Transcript evaluations	• 95.5% reported crash or near-miss during past year while driving home after night shift. • No job performance effects reported with consistent sleep and wake patterns. • Many nurses reported that changing from night work to day activities was fatiguing and affected performance.
Tucker et al. 1998a	862 workers from 17 manufacturing companies divided into four groups depending on start time and shift length: • 98% male • Age M 41.4 • United Kingdom	• One-time administration of *Survey of Shiftwork* (SOS): ○ 12-h day starting at 6 a.m. ○ 8-h day starting at 6 a.m. ○ 12-h day starting at 7 a.m. ○ 8-h day starting at 7 a.m. • All rapid forward or backward rotations • Work about 45 h/wk	One-time administration: *Survey of Shiftwork* (SOS) to measure cardiovascular disease, musculoskeletal pain, fatigue	• ANCOVA • Covariates: age; dependents; years on shift work; time on present system; work hours; workload; control of work pacing; sleep need	• Compared to 8-h shifts, 12-h shifts showed less symptoms of chronic fatigue (p < 0.05), more cardiovascular symptoms (p < 0.05), and more symptoms of musculoskeletal pain (p < 0.001) • 12-h shifts with early changeover showed more cardiovascular problems (p < 0.01) and musculoskeletal pain (p < 0.001); fatigue symptoms were NS. • 8-h rotation with late changeover showed fewest physical symptoms.

Abbreviations used: BMI = body mass index; BP = blood pressure; CI = 95% confidence interval; CIR = cumulative incidence ratio; D = day; E = evening; h = hours; M = mean; N = night; NS = significant; OR = odds ratio; PR = prevalence risk ratio; R = range; RR = relative risk ratio; wk = week; y = years. ¹omb reference appears also in Table 7.

3.3b Extended Work Shifts Combined with More than 40-Hours Work per Week and Injuries

Mitchell and Williamson [2000] reported that injury data from Australian electrical power station workers were similar after changing from an 8-hour shift to a 12-hour shift; two injuries occurred during the 8-hour schedule, and one occurred during the 12-hour schedule.

3.3c Extended Work Shifts Combined with More than 40-Hours Work per Week and Health Behaviors

Mitchell and Williamson [2000] reported that 47% of workers on an 8-hour 3-shift weekly rotation reported using alcohol as a sleep aid when compared with 17% of workers on a 12-hour fast rotation. The 8-hour shifts also had a higher percentage of workers smoking.

3.3d Extended Work Shifts Combined with More than 40-Hours Work per Week and Performance

Four studies reported some deterioration in performance when 12-hour shifts were combined with more than 40 hours work per week. Novak and Auvil-Novak [1996] reported an unexpected outcome from the focus groups of nurses who worked four 12-hour night shifts per week: nearly all nurses reported an automobile crash or near-miss during the previous 12 months while driving home after working a 12-hour night shift. The nurses reported no job performance effects when they maintained consistent sleep and wake times, but changing from night work to day activities was fatiguing and affected performance. In a field study, Fischer et al. [2000] examined the 2nd, 6th, and 10th hours of 12-hour shifts in Brazilian petrochemical plant workers and reported a significant decline in subjective alertness at the 10th hour for both day and night shifts. Similarly, Mitchell and Williamson [2000] reported more vigilance task errors at the end of

12-hour day and night shifts when compared to the beginning of the shifts in Australian power plant workers, while no effect was reported for an 8-hour schedule. On the other hand, significant improvements were observed for simple reaction time and grammatical reasoning tests given at the end of the 12-hour shift when compared to the beginning. Although Duchon et al. [1997] reported no differences between 8- and 12-hour shifts on cognitive and psychomotor performance in Canadian mine workers, the heart rate findings suggest that the 12-hour workers slowed the pace of their work.

3.4 FINDINGS ASSOCIATED WITH VERY LONG SHIFTS

Three studies examined the relationship between very long shifts and immune function or performance. The studies were conducted in Ireland, Japan, and New Zealand. Table 9 displays the methods and results for the studies that examined very long work shifts.

3.4a Very Long Shifts and Other Illnesses

Nakano et al. [1998] reported better immune function in drivers who were allowed to work overtime as compared with drivers having work-hour restrictions. This Japanese study examined taxi drivers working 48-hour or longer shifts in 1992 and again in 1993, before and during the economic depression.

3.4b Very Long Shifts and Performance

A study in Ireland by Leonard et al. [1998] reported declines in two tests of alertness and concentration in medical residents who had worked 32-hour on-call shifts. They reported no significant declines in a test of psychomotor performance or a test of memory. A New Zealand survey of anesthesiologists linked long working hours to self-reported clinical errors [Gander et al. 2000].

Table 9. Studies Examining Very Long Work Shifts: Methods and Findings

Author, Date	Sample	Description of Very Long Work Shift	Health or Safety Measure	Statistical Methods Controls	Results Reported By Authors
Gander et al. 2000	• 301 anesthetists: ◦ Specialists M age 46 ◦ Trainees M age 33 ◦ Gender not reported • New Zealand	One-time questionnaire (how many hours can work safely): • Maximum h/wk • Ongoing h/wk	One-time questionnaire: self-reported fatigue-related errors during last 6 months	Logistic regression	Specialists exceeding self-report limits on work hours increased the risk for fatigue-related errors in the last six months by 1.37 (CI 1.14 – 1.65) to 1.48 (CI 1.21 – 1.8).
Leonard et al. 1998	• 16 junior pre-registration medical house officers: • Men 50% • Age R 23 – 28; • Ireland	• Compared: ◦ Pre-call shift (8 – 10-h) ◦ Long, 32-h on-call shift • Randomly assigned order shifts tested	• Tests: Delayed Recall, Critical Flicker Fusion, Trail-making, Stroop Color Word Test, Grammatical Reasoning • Tested at end of one shift (4 – 6 p.m.)	Wilcoxon matched pairs	• End of 32-h on-call shift showed deterioration ($p < .05$) on median scores of alertness and concentration tests (Stroop Color Word Test, Trail-making Test). • No significant differences reported on Delayed Story Recall, Critical Flicker Fusion, or Grammatical Reasoning Tests.
Nakano et al. 1998	Random sample of 101 male taxi drivers: • Age R 40 – 59 • Japan	Examined company records in 1992 – 1993: • 48 h shifts started at 6 – 8 a.m. and ended at 2 a.m. next day with 1 day off/week. • Group A allowed to work past 2 a.m. for overtime. Group B not allowed overtime.	In 1992 and 1993 tested blood mononuclear cell proliferation assay and induction of Th1-type (IL-2) and Th2-type (IL-4) cytokines.	Student t-tests	During economic depression (1993), group B (not allowed overtime) increased IL-4 production and showed more depressed lymphocyte proliferation response than group A, who was allowed to work overtime.

Note. Abbreviations used: BMI = body mass index; BP = blood pressure; CI = 95% confidence interval; CIR = cumulative incidence ratio; D = day; E = evening; h = hours; M = mean; N = night; NS = not significant; OR = odds ratio; PR = prevalence risk ratio; R = range; RR = relative risk ratio; wk = week; y = year

Overtime was associated with poorer perceived general health, increased injury rates, more illnesses, or increased mortality in 16 of 22 studies.

4. Summary

4.1 OVERTIME

Overtime was associated with poorer perceived general health, increased injury rates, more illnesses, or increased mortality in 16 of 22 studies. One meta-analysis of long work hours suggested a possible weak relationship with preterm birth. Overtime was associated with unhealthy weight gain in two studies, increased alcohol use in two of three studies, increased smoking in one of two studies, and poorer neuropsychological test performance in one study. Some reports did not support this trend, finding no relationship between long work hours and leisure-time physical activity in two of three studies and no relationship with drug abuse in one study.

4.2 EXTENDED WORK SHIFTS

A pattern of deteriorating performance on psychophysiological tests and injuries while working long hours was observed across study findings, particularly in very long shifts and when 12-hour shifts were combined with more than 40 hours of work a week. Four studies reported that the 9th to 12th hours of work were associated with feelings of decreased alertness and increased fatigue, lower cognitive function, declines in vigilance on task measures, or increased injuries. Effects after the 12th hour of work were not examined. Two studies examining physicians working very long shifts reported deterioration in various measures of cognitive performance.

When 12-hour shifts were combined with other work-related demands, a pattern of more adverse findings was detected across studies. Six studies, examining 12-hour shifts combined with more than 40 hours of work per week, reported increases in health complaints, deterioration in performance, or slower pace of work. Two studies that compared 8- and 12-hour schedules during day and night shifts reported that 12-hour night shifts were associated with more fatigue, smoking, or alcohol use. Two studies examining start times for 12-hour shifts reported that decrements in alertness or more health complaints were associated with early 6:00 a.m. start times. One study examining 12-hour shifts in hot work environments also reported a slower pace of work as compared to shorter shifts. Another study examining high workloads during 12-hour shifts showed increased discomfort and deterioration in performance as compared to shorter shifts.

More definitive statements about differences between 8-hour and 12-hour shifts are difficult due to the inconsistencies in work schedules examined across studies. Work schedules differed by the time of day (i.e., day, evening, night), fixed versus rotating schedules, speed of rotation, direction of rotation, number of hours worked per week, number of consecutive days worked, and number of rest days on weekends. All of these factors can influence how overtime relates to health and safety. In addition, some studies of extended work shifts did not report how many hours participants worked per week or other details about their work schedules, which may have accounted for the findings. Also, some studies reported findings for groups of workers working mixed directional shift rotations and varying numbers of hours per week, details which complicated an assessment of the results.

4.3 OTHER WORK SCHEDULE CHARACTERISTICS

Few studies examined the combined influence of shift work and overtime on health. The laboratory study by Rosa et al. [1998] reported that four 12-hour night shifts per week were associated with the highest upper extremity muscle fatigue as compared to five 8-hour days and four 12-hour days. Trinkoff and Storr [1998] reported that nurses on extended night or extended rotating shifts were at increased odds for alcohol use and that extended night shifts increased the odds for smoking.

Some findings indicated that worker ability to exert control over work schedules may have influenced outcomes. For example, Smith et al. [1998] reported that 12-hour shifts having some flexibility in start times were associated with more favorable sleep quality, psychological well-being, and alertness, as compared with rigid schedules. One of the 52 summarized studies directly examined the influence of mandated or involuntary overtime. The combined influence of high pressure to work overtime and low rewards was associated by van der Hulst and Geurts [2001] with an increased risk for somatic complaints, poor recovery, burnout, and negative work-home interference. Previously published reviews of the literature did not address the influence of mandated overtime on health and safety [Rosa 1995; Sparks et al. 1997; Spurgeon et al. 1997]. Golden and Jorgensen [2002], however, cautioned that the mandated nature of overtime may limit the worker's ability to plan for sleep and recuperation, and to arrange for child care and other family responsibilities. As a result, health and safety effects associated with mandated versus voluntary overtime may differ.

4.4 COMPENSATION, VACATION TIME, COMMUTE TIME

Siu and Donald [1995] and van der Hulst and Geurts [2001] suggested that compensation may reduce adverse effects. In addition, Nakano et al. [1998] indicated that economic conditions (prosperity as compared with recession or depression) may influence the relationship between pay, overtime, and health and safety. Few studies, however, systematically examined how compensation influenced the relationship between long work hours and health and safety.

Length of vacation and commute time may also influence associations of overtime with health and safety. Higher numbers of annual leave days may allow more rest and may reduce the impact of overtime. Also, commute time to work may add to the job strain and may influence associations with overtime. Few studies have examined the influence of vacation time or commute time on long work hours and health.

4.5 GENDER AND AGE

Studies have given more attention to male workers than to female workers and less is known about how overtime and extended work shifts influence health and safety in women. Statistics Canada [2000] reported that women tend to spend more of their time away from work on child care and domestic responsibilities, which may reduce the time available for sleep and recovery from work. The study by Fredriksson et al. [1999] provided some support for increased risk for musculoskeletal disorders when long hours worked combined with additional domestic workload.

Another consideration is the influence of long work hours on reproductive outcomes. One meta-analysis reported a possible weak relationship between overtime and preterm births, and another study reported an association between long work hours and subfecundity [Mozurkewich et al. 2000; Tuntiseranee et al. 1998]. Few studies have examined the influence of overtime and extended work shifts in pregnant women, or prenatal and neonatal mortality and morbidity, as well as fertility rates.

One laboratory study examining the influence of age on extended work shifts reported that younger participants maintained better performance across extended work shifts when compared with older participants [Reid and Dawson 2001]. However, few studies have examined the effect of worker age on performance or health and safety in real-work environments. In addition, little is known about the way various work tasks and other work-related factors influence the relationship with age.

4.6 CHRONIC HEALTH PROBLEMS

Studies of long working hours have examined healthy workers for the risk of contracting an acute myocardial infarction, diabetes mellitus, hypertension, subfecundity, and preterm birth. Little data, however, are available about symptom management and disease progression in workers with pre-existing chronic conditions.

According to Yelin et al. [1999], the 1992 data from the U.S. Health and Retirement Survey indicated that 83% of all persons aged 51 to 61 years live with a self-reported chronic condition.

4.7 OCCUPATIONAL EXPOSURES

Two of the 52 summarized reports addressed occupational exposures (i.e., chemical, heat, noise, lifting) in conjunction with overtime and extended work shifts. Mizoue et al. [2001] reported that overtime was associated with more sick building syndrome symptoms, and Brake and Bates [2001] found that miners working long shifts in hot environments paced themselves, thus, reducing their effort. Little has been reported on other occupational exposures. Extended work shifts and overtime lengthen exposure times and shorten recovery times, and the health consequences are uncertain.

> Few studies have examined how long working hours influence health and safety outcomes in older workers, women, persons with pre-existing health problems, and workers with hazardous occupational exposures.

5. Concluding Remarks

The number of published studies examining overtime and extended work shifts appears to be increasing. Recent reviews that address overtime include approximately 34 research reports published over a span of about 32 years [Sparks et al. 1997; Spurgeon et al. 1997]. In comparison, the current search for reports published during the past 8 years found 75 reports that examined overtime, extended work shifts, or very long shifts. The latest review of long work hours by van der Hulst [2003] includes an additional 13 studies that have been published since 1996.

Despite the increased current interest in long working hours, research questions remain about the ways overtime and extended work shifts influence health and safety. Few studies have examined how the number of hours worked per week, shift work, shift length, the degree of control over one's work schedule, compensation for overtime, and other characteristics of work schedules interact and relate to health and safety. Few studies have examined how long working hours influence health and safety outcomes in older workers, women, persons with pre-existing health problems, and workers with hazardous occupational exposures.

Previous research indicates that the influence of overtime and extended work shifts on health and safety may involve a complex interaction of several work schedule characteristics, as well as work tasks, worker characteristics, compensation, commute time, occupational exposures, and nature of worker control over work schedules. As a consequence, future research would benefit from a clear and complete description of the work schedules and other factors mentioned in this document. Such an approach would facilitate a detailed comparison of findings across studies.

> Few studies have examined how number of hours worked per week, shift work, shift length, the degree of control over one's work schedule, compensation for overtime, and other characteristics of work schedules interact and relate to health and safety.

References

Åkerstedt T, Fredlund P, Gillberg M, Jansson B [2002]. A prospective study of fatal occupational accidents—relationship to sleeping difficulties and occupational factors. J Sleep Res *11*(1):69–71.

Åkerstedt T, Kecklund G, Gillberg M, Lowden A, Axelsson J [2000]. Sleepiness and days of recovery. Transportation Research Part F: Traffic Psy Behaviour *3*(4):251–261 ‡.

Araki Y, Muto, and Asakura T. [1999]. Psychosomatic symptoms of Japanese working women and their need for stress management. Ind Health *37*(2):253–262 ‡.

Axelsson J, Kecklund G, Åkerstedt T, Lowden A [1998]. Effects of alternating 8- and 12-hour shifts on sleep, sleepiness, physical effort and performance. Scand J Work Environ Health *24* Suppl 3:62–68.

Bergqvist U, Wolgast E, Nilsson B, Voss M [1995]. Musculoskeletal disorders among visual display terminal workers: individual, ergonomic, and work organizational factors. Ergonomics *38*(4):763–776.

Bliese PD, Halverson RR [1996]. Individual and nomothetic models of job stress: an examination of work hours, cohesion, and well-being. J Appl Soc Psychol *26*(13): 1171–1189 ‡.

Brake DJ, Bates GP [2001]. Fatigue in industrial workers under thermal stress on extended shift lengths. Occup Med (Oxford) *51*(7):456–463.

Defoe DM, Power ML, Holzman GB, Carpentieri A, Schulkin J [2001]. Long hours and little sleep: work schedules of residents in obstetrics and gynecology. Obstet Gynecol *97*(6):1015–1018 ‡.

Duchon JC, Smith TJ, Keran CM, Koehler EJ [1997]. Psychophysiological manifestations of performance during work on extended workshifts. Int J Ind Ergon *20*(1):39–49.

Ettner SL, Grzywacz JG [2001]. Workers' perceptions of how jobs affect health: A social ecological perspective. J Occup Health Psychol *6*(2):113.

Fischer FM, Moreno CRD, Borges FND, Louzada FM [2000]. Implementation of 12-hour shifts in a Brazilian petrochemical plant: impact on sleep and alertness. Chronobiol Int *17*(4):521–537.

Fredriksson K, Alfredsson L, Köster M, Thorbjörnsson CB, Toomingas A, Torgén M, Kilbom A [1999]. Risk factors for neck and upper limb disorders: results from 24 years of follow up. Occup Environ Med 56(1):59–66.

Gander PH, Merry A, Millar MM, Weller J [2000]. Hours of work and fatigue-related error: a survey of New Zealand anaesthetists. Anaesth Intensive Care 28(2):178–183.

Gillberg M [1998]. Subjective alertness and sleep quality in connection with permanent 12-hour day and night shifts. Scand J Work Environ Health *24* Suppl 3:76–80 ‡.

‡ indicates paper not discussed in this document.

Golden L, Jorgensen H [2002]. Economic Policy Institute briefing paper: time after time mandatory over-time in the U.S. economy. Retrieved 1/13/02 from <http://epinet.org>.

Hänecke K, Tiedemann S, Nachreiner F, Grzech-Šukalo H [1998]. Accident risk as a function of hour at work and time of day as determined from accident data and exposure models for the German working population. Scand J Work Environ Health *24* Suppl 3:43–48.

Hayashi T, Kobayashi Y, Yamaoka K, Yano E [1996]. Effect of overtime work on 24-hour ambulatory blood pressure. J Occup Environ Med *38*(10):1007–1011.

Hetrick R [2000]. Analyzing the recent upward surge in overtime hours. Monthly Labor Rev *123*(2):30–33.

International Labour Office [2002]. Key indicators of the labour market. Retrieved February 13, 2002, from <http://www.ilo.org/public/english/employment/strat/kilm/trends.htm#figure%206b>.

International Labour Office [2003]. Key indicators of the labour market 2001–2002, Palm Version. Available from Routledge/Taylor & Francis, New York.

Ishizaki M, Martikainen P, Nakagawa H, Marmot M, Japan Work Stress and Health Cohort Study Group. [2001]. Socioeconomic status, workplace characteristics and plasma fibrinogen level of Japanese male employees. Scand J Work Environ Health *27*(4):287–291 ‡.

Iskra-Golec I, Folkard S, Marek T, Noworol C [1996]. Health, well-being and burnout of ICU nurses on 12- and 8-h shifts. Work Stress *10*(3):251–256 ‡.

Iwasaki K, Sasaki T, Oka T, Hisanaga N [1998]. Effect of working hours on biological functions related to cardiovascular system among salesmen in a machinery manufacturing company. Ind Health *36*:361–367.

Johnson MD, Sharit J [2001]. Impact of a change from an 8-h to a 12-h shift schedule on workers and occupational injury rates. Int J Ind Ergon *27*(5):303–319.

Kageyama T, Nishikido N, Kobayashi T, Kurokawa Y, Kaneko T, Kabuto M [1998]. Long commuting time, extensive overtime, and sympathodominant state assessed in terms of short-term heart rate variability among male white-collar workers in the Tokyo megalopolis. Ind Health *36*(3):209–217.

Kageyama T, Nishikido N, Kobayashi T, Kawagoe H [2001]. Estimated sleep debt and work stress in Japanese white-collar workers. Psychiatr Clin Neurosci *55*:217–219.

Kaliterna L, Prizmic Z [1998]. Evaluation of the survey of shiftworkers (SOS) short version of the stan-dard shiftwork index. Int J Ind Ergon *21*(3-4):259–265 ‡.

Kawakami N, Araki S, Takatsuka N, Shimizu H, Ishibashi H [1999]. Overtime, psychosocial working con-ditions, and occurrence of non-insulin dependent diabetes mellitus in Japanese men. J Epidemiol Community Health *53*(6):359–363.

‡ indicates paper not discussed in this document.

Kirkcaldy BD, Levine R, Shephard RJ [2000]. The impact of working hours on physical and psychological health of German managers. Eur Rev Appl Psychol *50*(4):443–449.

Kirkcaldy BD, Trimpop R, Cooper CL [1997]. Working hours, job stress, work satisfaction, and accident rates among medical practitioners and allied personnel. Int J Stress Manag *4*(2):79–87.

Knauth P [1998]. Innovative worktime arrangements. Scand J Work Environ Health *24* (Suppl 3):13–17.

Kundi M, Koller M, Stefan H, Lehner L, Kaindlsdorfer S, Rottenbücher S [1995]. Attitudes of nurses towards 8-h and 12-h shift systems. Work Stress *9*(2-3):134–139 ‡.

Leonard C, Fanning N, Attwood J, Buckley M [1998]. The effect of fatigue, sleep deprivation and onerous working hours on the physical and mental wellbeing of pre-registration house officers. Ir J Med Sci *167*(1):22–25.

Lipscomb JA, Trinkoff AM, Geiger-Brown J, Brady B [2002]. Work-schedule characteristics and reported musculoskeletal disorders of registered nurses. Scand J Work Environ Health *28*(6): 394–401.

Liu Y, Tanaka H, The Fukuoka Heart Study Group [2002]. Overtime work, insufficient sleep, and risk of non-fatal acute myocardial infarction in Japanese men. Occup Environ Med *59*(7):447–451.

Lowden A, Kecklund G, Axelsson J, Åkerstedt T [1998]. Change from an 8-hour shift to a 12-hour shift, attitudes, sleep, sleepiness and performance. Scand J Work Environ Health *24* Suppl 3:69–75.

Lowery JT, Borgerding JA, Zhen B, Glazner JE, Bondy J, Kreiss K [1998]. Risk factors for injury among construction workers at Denver International Airport. Am J Ind Med *34*(2):113–120.

Macdonald W, Bendak S [2000]. Effects of workload level and 8- versus 12-h workday duration on test battery performance. Int J Ind Ergon *26*(3):399–416.

Macias DJ, Hafner J, Brillman JC, Tandberg D [1996]. Effect of time of day and duration into shift on hazardous exposures to biological fluids. Acad Emerg Med *3*(6):605–610.

Maruyama S, Morimoto K [1996]. Effects of long workhours on life-style, stress and quality of life among intermediate Japanese managers. Scand J Work Environ Health *22*(5):353–359 ‡.

Mitchell RJ, Williamson AM [2000]. Evaluation of an 8-hour versus a 12-hour shift roster on employees at a power station. Appl Ergon *31*(1):83–93.

Mitler MM, Miller JC, Lipsitz JJ, Walsh JK, Wylie CD [1997]. The sleep of long-haul truck drivers. N Engl J Med *337*(11):755–61 ‡.

Mizoue T, Reijula K, Andersson K [2001]. Environmental tobacco smoke exposure and overtime work as risk factors for sick building syndrome in Japan. Am J Epidemiol *154*(9):803–808.

‡ indicates paper not discussed in this document.

Mozurkewich EL, Luke B, Avni M, Wolf FM [2000]. Working conditions and adverse pregnancy outcome: a meta-analysis. Obstet Gynecol *95*(4):623–635.

Murray A, Safran DG, Rogers WH, Inui T, Chang H, Montgomery JE [2000]. Part-time physicians. Physician workload and patient-based assessments of primary care performance. Arch Fam Med *9*(4):327–332 ‡.

Nakamura K, Shimai S, Kikuchi S, Takahashi H, Tanaka M, Nakano S, Motohashi Y, Nakadaira H, Yamamoto M [1998]. Increases in body mass index and waist circumference as outcomes of working overtime. Occup Med (Lond) *48*(3):169–173.

Nakanishi N, Nishina K, Yoshida H, Matsuo Y, Nagano K, Nakamura K, Suzuki K, Tatara K [2001a]. Hours of work and the risk of developing impaired fasting glucose or type 2 diabetes mellitus in Japanese male office workers. Occup Environ Med *58*(9):569–574.

Nakanishi N, Yoshida H, Nagano K, Kawashimo H, Nakamura K, Tatara K [2001b]. Long working hours and risk for hypertension in Japanese male white collar workers. J Epidemiol Community Health *55*(5):316–322.

Nakano Y, Nakamura S, Hirata M, Harada K, Ando K, Tabuchi T, Matunaga I, Oda H [1998]. Immune function and lifestyle of taxi drivers in Japan. Ind Health *36*(1):32–39.

Novak RD, Auvil-Novak SE [1996]. Focus group evaluation of night nurse shiftwork difficulties and coping strategies. Chronobiol Int *13*(6):457–463.

Nylén L, Voss M, Floderus B [2001]. Mortality among women and men relative to unemployment, part-time work, overtime work, and extra work: a study based on data from the Swedish Twin Registry. Occup Environ Med *58*(1):52–57.

Ognianova VM, Dalbokova DL, Stanchev V [1998]. Stress states, alertness and individual differences under 12-hour shiftwork. Int J Ind Ergon *21*(3–4), 283–291 ‡.

Paley MJ, Price JM, Tepas DI [1998]. The impact of a change in rotating shift schedules: a comparison of the effects of 8, 10 and 14 h work shifts. Int J Ind Ergon *21*(3–4):293–305 ‡.

Park J, Kim Y, Cho Y, Woo KH, Chung HK, Iwasaki K, Oka T, Sasaki T, Hisanaga N [2001a]. Regular overtime and cardiovascular functions. Ind Health *39*(3):244–249.

Park J, Kim Y, Chung HK, Hisanaga N [2001b]. Long working hours and subjective fatigue symptoms. Ind Health *39*(3):250–254.

Proctor SP, White RF, Robins TG, Echeverria D, Rocskay AZ [1996]. Effect of overtime work on cognitive function in automotive workers. Scand J Work Environ Health *22*(2):124–132.

‡ indicates paper not discussed in this document.

Prunier-Poulmaire S, Gadbois C, Volkoff S [1998]. Combined effects of shift systems and work requirements on customs officers. Scand J Work Environ Health *24* Suppl 3:134–140.

Reid K, Dawson D [2001]. Comparing performance on a simulated 12-hour shift rotation in young and older subjects. Occup Environ Med *58*(1):58–62.

Ribet C, Derriennic F [1999]. Age, working conditions, and sleep disorders: a longitudinal analysis in the French cohort E.S.T.E.V. Sleep *22*(4):491–504 ‡.

Rones PL, Iig RE, Gardner JM [1997]. Trends in hours of work since the mid-1970s. Monthly Labor Rev *120*(4):3–14.

Rosa RR [1995]. Extended workshifts and excessive fatigue. J Sleep Res *4* (Suppl. 2):51–56.

Rosa RR, Bonnet MH, Cole LL [1998]. Work schedule and task factors in upper-extremity fatigue. Hum Factors *40*(1):150–158.

Schroeder DJ, Rosa RR, Witt LA [1998]. Some effects of 8- vs. 10-hour work schedules on the test performance/alertness of air traffic control specialists. Int J Ind Ergon *21*:307–321.

Shields M [1999]. Long working hours and health. Health Rep *11*(2):33–48.

Simpson CL, Severson RK [2000]. Risk of injury in African American hospital workers. J Occup Environ Med *42*(10):1035–1040.

Siu O-L, Donald I [1995]. Psychosocial factors at work and workers' health in Hong Kong: an exploratory study. Bulletin of the Hong Kong Psychological Society *34/35*:30–56.

Smith L, Totterdell P, Folkard S [1995]. Shiftwork effects in nuclear power workers: A field study using portable computers. Work Stress *9*(2-3):235–244.

Smith L, Hammond T, Macdonald I, Folkard S [1998]. 12-h shifts are popular but are they a solution? Int J Ind Ergon *21*(3-4):323–331.

Sokejima S, Kagamimori S [1998]. Working hours as a risk factor for acute myocardial infarction in Japan: case-control study. Br Med J *317*(7161):775–780.

Sparks K, Cooper CL, Fried Y, Shirom A [1997]. The effects of hours of work on health: a meta-analytic review. J Occup Organ Psychol *70*(4):391–408.

Spurgeon A, Harrington JM, Cooper CL [1997]. Health and safety problems associated with long working hours: a review of the current position. Occup Environ Med *54*(6):367–375.

Statistics Canada [2000]. Women in Canada 2000: a gender-based statistical report. Ottawa, Can: Statistics Canada, pp. 89–503–XPE.

‡ indicates paper not discussed in this document.

Steele MT, Ma OJ, Watson WA, Thomas HA [2000]. Emergency medicine residents' shiftwork tolerance and preference. Acad Emerg Med 7(6):670–673 ‡.

Suskin N, Ryan G, Fardy J, Clarke H, McKelvie R [1998]. Clinical workload decreases the level of aerobic fitness in housestaff physicians. J Cardiopulm Rehabil 18(3):216–220 ‡.

Takahashi M, Arito H, Fukuda H [1999a]. Nurses' workload associated with 16-h night shifts. II: effects of a nap taken during the shifts. Psychiatr Clin Neurosci 53(2):223–225.

Takahashi M, Fukuda H, Miki K, Haratani T, Kurabayashi L, Hisanaga N, Arito H, Takahashi H, Egoshi M, Sakurai M [1999b]. Shift work-related problems in 16-h night shift nurses (2): effects on subjective symptoms, physical activity, heart rate, and sleep. Ind Health 37(2):228–236 ‡.

Trinkoff AM, Storr CL [1998]. Work schedule characteristics and substance use in nurses. Am J Ind Med 34(3):266–271 ‡.

Tucker P, Barton J, Folkard S [1996]. Comparison of eight and 12 hour shifts: impacts on health, wellbeing, and alertness during the shift. Occup Environ Med 53(11):767–772 ‡.

Tucker P, Smith L, Macdonald I, Folkard S [1998a]. The impact of early and late shift changeovers on sleep, health, and well-being in 8- and 12-hour shift systems. J Occup Health Psychol 3(3):265–275.

Tucker P, Smith L, Macdonald I, Folkard S [1998b]. Shift length as a determinant of retrospective on-shift alertness. Scand J Work Environ Health 24 Suppl 3:49–54.

Tucker P, Smith L, Macdonald I, Folkard S [1999]. Distribution of rest days in 12-hour shift systems: impacts on health, wellbeing, and on shift alertness. Occup Environ Med 56(3):206–214 ‡.

Tuntiseranee P, Olsen J, Geater A, Kor-anantakul O [1998]. Are long working hours and shiftwork risk factors for subfecundity? A study among couples from southern Thailand. Occup Environ Med 55(2):99–105.

van der Hulst M [2003]. Long workhours and health. Scand J Work Environ Health 29:171–188.

van der Hulst M, Geurts S [2001]. Associations between overtime and psychological health in high and low reward jobs. Work Stress 15(3):227–240.

Voss M, Floderus B, Diderichsen F [2001]. Physical, psychosocial, and organizational factors relative to sickness absence: a study based on Sweden Post. Occup Environ Med 58(3):178–184.

Worrall L, Cooper CL [1999]. Working patterns and working hours: their impact on UK managers. Leadersh Organ Dev J 20(1):6–10.

Yelin EH, Trupin LS, Sebesta DS [1999]. Transitions in employment, morbidity, and disability among persons ages 51-61 with musculoskeletal and non-musculoskeletal conditions in the U.S., 1992-1994. Arthritis Rheum 42(4):769–779.

‡ indicates paper not discussed in this document.

Additional References

Rosa RR, Colligan MJ [1997]. Plain language about shiftwork. Cincinnati, OH: Department of Health and Human Services, Public Health Service, Centers for Disease Control and Prevention, National Institute for Occupational Safety and Health, Division of Biomedical and Behavioral Science, DHHS (NIOSH) Publication No. 97-145.

Sauter SS, Brightwell WS, Colligan MJ, Hurrell JJ Jr, Katz TM, LeGrande DE, Lessin N, Lippin RA, Lipscomb JA, Murphy LR, Peters RH, Keita GP, Robertson SR, Stellman JM, Swanson NG, Tetrick LE [2002]. The changing organization of work and the safety and health of working people. Cincinnati, OH: Department of Health and Human Services, Public Health Service, Centers for Disease Control and Prevention, National Institute for Occupational Safety and Health, Division of Applied Research and Technology, DHHS (NIOSH) Publication No. 2002-116.